RUNES

IN 10 MINUTES

Other Avon Books by
R. T. Kaser

I CHING IN TEN MINUTES
TAROT IN TEN MINUTES

RUNES
IN 10 MINUTES

R. T. KASER

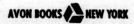
AVON BOOKS · NEW YORK

SCRABBLE® is a registered trademark of Hasbro, Inc.© 1993. Milton Bradley Company is a division of Hasbro, Inc. All rights reserved. Used with permission.

RUNES IN 10 MINUTES is an original publication of Avon Books. This work has never before appeared in book form.

AVON BOOKS
A division of
The Hearst Corporation
1350 Avenue of the Americas
New York, New York 10019

Copyright © 1995 by Richard T. Kaser
Rune illustrations for "Wild Bill's Vision Quest" by William B. Cox, based on a concept by R. T. Kaser. Copyright © 1993, 1994.
"RTKRunes" fonts copyright © 1993 by R. T. Kaser
Published by arrangement with the author
Library of Congress Catalog Card Number: 94-47407
ISBN: 0-380-77605-7

Library of Congress Cataloging in Publication Data:

Kaser, R. T.
  Runes in 10 minutes / R. T. Kaser.
    p. cm.
Includes bibliographical references and index.
1. Magic 2. Runes—Miscellanea. 3. Fortune-telling by runes.
I. Title. II. Title: Runes in ten minutes.
BF1623.R89K37 1995   94-47407
133.3'3—dc20   CIP

First Avon Books Trade Printing: April 1995

AVON TRADEMARK REG. U.S. PAT. OFF. AND IN OTHER COUNTRIES, MARCA REGISTRADA, HECHO EN U.S.A.

Printed in the U.S.A.

OPM 10 9 8 7 6 5 4 3 2 1

For all the kith and kinfolk
and with love
to
Mom and Dad

GIBU AUJA
I give good luck

— Inscription on an ancient amulet

PREFACE

Runes are the enchanted—and enchanting!—alphabet used by our European ancestors . . . to write their names on things . . . to read the future into things . . . and to try to gain control over things.

Runes look like this: 🄿🅄🄵🄿🅁🄺 . . . . Within ten minutes, you'll be using these charming letter tiles as tools for dealing with your own life in your own way.

Or, what the hay, if you'd rather work with your everyday ABC's, be my guest: 🄰🄱🄲🄳🄴🄵🄶 . . . . Scrabble® tiles work just great. Go get your set, I'll wait.

Of course, it's also fun to make your own Runes, and *Runes in Ten Minutes* is full of tips for creating a set of your own. All you *really* need to get started is a scratch pad and a pen. Write one letter of the alphabet—or one Rune—on each square of paper and you're ready to begin.

Using your Runes is as easy as 1, 2, 3. . . .

1   Just come up with your question or issue.

2   Mix up your Runes (or alphabet tiles), and select a few from the pile.

3   Read meaning into the Runes you have drawn. Interpret your answers.

Using *Runes in Ten Minutes*, interpreting your Runes is also quite easy. Just turn to the Answer section for the chapter (Reading) you are doing at the time, or consult the Master Answer section at the back of the book.

That's all there is to it.

But to tell you the whole truth, <u>you don't even need a set of Runes</u> or a pile of alphabet tiles to have fun with this book.

You can learn a lot about yourself by just using the letters in your name or the numbers in your birthday to look up Runes. To take this route, start with Reading #4. Then go on to Readings #5, #6, #7, #10, #11, #12, #13, #20, #21, #22, and #23. Going at it this way, you'll have a chance to see if Runes are for you before you invest your time or money in a set.

But if you'd really like to experience a bit of the "magic" your ancestors must have felt when, of an evening, they sat by the campfire wondering which route would be best to take at sunrise . . . a set of Runes is the only way to go.

Let me say it simply—for we've only got about eight minutes left—there is something *magical* about the way the Runes feel tumbling through your hands as you mix them up . . .

There is something *mysterious* about the way one Rune will invariably be drawn into your palm . . .

There is something *wonderful* about the moment when you look to see which Rune you have drawn, and . . .

There is something *uncanny* about the answers that come.

If you want to get started with the book, I won't keep you but another minute. The only thing left for you to do at this point is decide which way you want to go. This book offers three routes.

- ■ Front to back
  For those who like to start things at the start, turn to the first chapter (Reading #1), and the book will take you by the hand and do the rest. You'll be using your Runes immediately to ask questions and get answers about yourself, your friends, and your family. Go on to the next Reading whenever you're ready to continue. There are 24 Readings in all, and lots of different things to do.

- ■ Back to front
  If you already have some experience with Runes—or if you'd just like to do your own thing—turn to Reading #24 and begin there. This Reading gives you the basics of using the Runes on your own. Once you ask your question and select your Runes, look up your answers in the Master Answer section at the back of the book.

■ All over the place
  Once you get the feel for how to use your Runes, you're
  welcome to scan the Contents or Index to see which questions you'd like to ask today. Just turn to that Reading and
  follow the instructions. You don't have to take the book
  in sequence if you don't want to. Jump around and experiment as your free spirit moves you.

If you're itching to get started, go for it now. But if you'd like to
know more about Runes before you begin, it will only take sixty seconds more. . . .

The Runes that appear in this book are the oldest known, esti-
mated by the British Museum to have been in use by A.D. 200.
Nobody knows how far back they actually go, but some say they
have their origin in the paintings on the walls of prehistoric caves.

Virtually all present-day Europeans used them at one time or
another, and, as a result, some Runic letters are to be found in the
modern alphabets of all the Romance languages. If your family originally came over on the boat from Italy; Germany, Austria, or
Switzerland; The Netherlands; Norway, Sweden, Finland, or
Denmark; England, Scotland, Wales . . . or even France and Spain,
the Runes are part of your heritage and birthright. But as a human
invention, they—of course—belong to the men and women of all
lands.

With the tools of the day—axes and knives—our primitive ancestors would consult the Runes by simply chopping off a tree limb,
hacking it into pieces, carving a letter of the Runic alphabet on
each slice, selecting a few at random, and taking these "lots" as
signs. When the evening's entertainment was done, Runes made
good fuel for the fire. It sounds relatively innocuous, all in all. But
what you have to remember is, our ancestors also believed. . . .

Plain and simply, they believed the Runes were *magic*. And there
is plenty going on within the Runes themselves to prove the point.
If you've got another minute, I'll tell you how the magic works.

Each Rune not only stood for a specific sound (just as each of our
modern letters does), but each Rune had a name that symbolized its
powers. And not only that, this name, you see, bore the same sound
as the letter of the alphabet it stood for. Wow! Talk about magic.
But wait, there's more. . . .

Even the order they come in was thought to be magical. As Norse legend has it, it took the god Odin nine long days and nights to set these Runic letters straight . . . thus unlocking their powers to work good deeds, bring good luck, and—greatest feat of all—bestow the gift of poetry upon mere mortals.

I could go on and on, but my time's up in about four minutes. Suffice it to say, so that you can have an authentic experience with the Runes, *Runes in Ten Minutes* tries to recapture not only the Runic method but a little of the magical feeling that rightfully belongs to this tradition. Here's how. . . .

Rather than translating the old Anglo-Saxon or Germanic names for each Rune into English—which often results in losing the sound of the original letter and thus a loss of the original "magic"—I have renamed the Runes so that their modern English names carry the same sound as the letter they represent. (Besides, they're easier to remember and relate to this way.)[1]

I've kept to the authentic ordering of the Runes (a sequence known as the Elder Futhark). That way, we can use the wisdom embedded in this highly ordered structure in the way it was designed and intended. You won't have to think about it very much, but many of the Readings in this book make use of the embedded structures to interpret your answers for you.

And thirdly—well, I'll let you be the judge, but I think the book just feels magical. Most of the Readings do at least two tricks—one described in the How To section, and the other in the Extra Credit section. Due to this "magical" construction, *Runes in Ten Minutes* actually offers you 48 different Readings to do. Sha-zam!

But is this system really magic?

For all the hocus-pocus and despite the mumbo jumbo in a few Rune books of late—I feel the Runes are largely about the *power of the word* to invoke images . . . evoke feelings . . . provoke emotions . . . and turn thought into action.

Runes in Ten Minutes puts this theory to the test as it guides you through a survey of your life, using the marvelously inventive Runes as the means to the noble ends of self-determination, self-realiza-

---

[1] But if you'd like to use the Anglo-Saxon names, they are covered in Readings #7, #8, #20, #21, #22, and #23, as well as in the Master Answer section of the Quick Reference Guide.

tion, self-actualization, self-fulfillment . . . whatever you want to call it.

The best thing to do at this point is to set you free with the book. But if you'd like to know why I wrote it—and what I learned about Runes in the process—it'll only take another minute or so.

When I sat down to craft *Runes in Ten Minutes*, I'd been dabbling with them for about ten years.[2] But I still found the various Runes hard to tell apart, their Anglo-Saxon names difficult to remember, and their meanings not very intuitively obvious. In short, Runes never felt very natural to me, when—ironically enough—with a name like Kaser, Runes ought to be in my blood.

My research—as usual—took me in a dozen directions at once. In my search for Runic knowledge, I had to read up on the Vikings, Etruscans, and Celts and on European mythology in general (fascinating stuff). I revisited *Grimm's Fairy Tales*, *The Poetic Edda*, and at one point, I got very interested in Pennsylvania Dutch hex signs.

But for all my readings on these many subjects, the thing that really helped me hit it off with the Runes was when I started to make them . . . out of slips of paper, sticks from the woods, stones from the shore, coins from my pocket . . . using pen, Swiss army knife, and, on occasion, electric jigsaw. An entire month was even spent at the computer, designing the Rune fonts for this book.[3] I had a blast.

As a result, *Runes in Ten Minutes* is full of craft projects (see the Extra, Extra Credit sections), which you can do if you like—and I highly recommend you try a couple. Because what I learned about Runes in the process of making them was: It's not only fun, but it's the most natural way to get to know, feel, and understand them.

All in all—and to make a long story shorter—I found the Runes to be a wonderfully spontaneous, even playful device.

But I should tell you—as a gentle parental warning, I guess—I also found Runes to be rather earthy. It only served to remind me of the forthright talk of the Amish farm boys I grew up with. It seemed right to me—even wholesome somehow—that Runes should be salt-of-the-earth kinds of things. So I let the Runes be Runes.

---

[2] Thanks to Ralph Blum.
[3] They were rendered using ALTSYS Fontographer V.4.0. for the Macintosh.

I was also often reminded of the folk sayings, traditional beliefs, and superstitions of the Swiss and German immigrants populating the little town I hail from. I saw in the Runes much consistency with the common sense, values, and folk wisdom of that rural community, whose people can trace themselves back to the same Swiss canton.[4] So forgive me, I may sound a little homespun sometimes. But that, too, seemed right for Runes.

At any rate—for I see my time is up—just let me say: By the time I got done writing this book, Runes had come to feel like second nature to me. I can only pray that I have managed to convey some small measure of this grand and glorious tradition of my humble ancestors.

What will it do for you?

Runes in Ten Minutes gives you the chance to recapture a little bit of our enchanted human past. But mostly, it puts the magical alphabet of the early Germanic tribes of Europe to work in helping you deal with everyday modern American life. By playing around with this book, you'll have an authentic experience with the Runes and you'll be well prepared to move on to more esoteric works on the subject.

Without further ado, then . . . I wish you best of luck in everything you choose to do, with—or without—the aid of these mere Runes.

— R. T. Kaser
Solar Eclipse
May 10, 1994

---

[4] For all those tuning in from Sugarcreek . . . I'll see you at the Swiss Festival.

CONTENTS

Contents

Contents

READ ME FIRST

This book presents a way of using the letters of the alphabet to think about things—past, present, and future. It works with "letter tiles," Ⓐ Ⓑ Ⓒ Ⓓ ... much like those found in that famous cross-word-puzzle game we all know and love. In fact, if you'd like to work with English letters, instead of the traditional Runic characters, be my guest! Your Scrabble® tiles will work just as well. (Just turn to Reading #1 to see which letter tiles you'll need from your set.)

The book also works with the authentic modern Rune sets sold in bookstores and catalogs, including the popular sets offered with books by Ralph Blum, Jason Cooper, and other authors—as well as with Rune cards, such as those by Donald Tyson.

To make your own set of Runes (within ten minutes!) consult the How To section of Reading #1. All you need is a scratch pad and a pencil. For other ways to make authentic Runes, see the Extra, Extra Credit sections throughout the book.

If you already own a set of Runes, they are most likely the same as the Runes used in this book, especially if you bought them in the United States. Check them against this list:

Some Rune sets substitute alternate characters for certain letters. If you own one of these sets, just make a mental note of which of your tiles is different. The answers in the book will still work fine. Common substitutions are:

ⓞ = ⓧ   ⓕ = ⓟ   ⓕ = ⓟ

TIPS

Keep your Runes in a bag or bowl—it not only keeps them neatly all in one place, but it's easy to select one simply by "drawing" it like a lottery number.

To use your Runes, the basic concept is simple. Just mix up your letter tiles while you think about the question or issue on your mind, then select a letter tile and look it up in the Answers.

Or you can take a handful of Runes, throw them on the floor, and then (without peeking) select a few to read (usually three).

To set the mood—light a candle, say a prayer, or take a few deep breaths to relax. Personal touches you can add: background music of your choice, a bowl of water, a stick of incense, a cloth to cast your Runes upon. Trouble concentrating? Take a walk or a hot bath.

Runes are best at answering "how" and "what" questions or dealing with issues. For help formulating questions, follow the instructions in each Reading's How To section or see Reading #24 for an overview, summary, and additional tips. Or browse the Index for a question that you'd like to ask today.

Once you've asked your question, select the Rune that simply comes into your hand. (You cannot do it wrong!) If you've cast your Runes on the floor, run your hand over the top of them and select the one that feels warm. Or just reach out and grab one from among all those you have cast.

Since the Runes are usually only depicted on one side of each tile, you may have to turn the tile over to see which Rune you have drawn. Turn the Rune over from side to side: � → ⊡ or ⬡ → Ⓐ, rather than from top to bottom: ⬡ ↓ ▣. Then look to see how your Rune has "fallen."

Sometimes you'll find that a Rune has fallen into your hand upside down: ▣ ⋒ ◁ ◁ ⋈ ▷ . . . . Since it's traditional to attach different meanings to upside-down Runes, many of the Readings in this book list separate answers for them. (If no upside-down Runes are listed, just ignore the reversed Runes for whatever activity you're doing at the time.)

It's also possible for a Rune to fall into your hand on its side: ▨ ▧ ▨ ▨ ▨ ▨ . . . or ▨ ▨ ▨ ▨ ▨ ▨ . By tradition, such Runes have no special meaning. Interpret those that fall "forward"

(⊡⊡⊡⊡⊡⊡) as upside-down Runes. Interpret those that fall "backward" (⊡⊡⊡⊡⊡⊡) as upright Runes. Or simply close your eyes and turn the Rune one way or the other.

Each Reading in the book is self-contained, but if you have questions about the methods or techniques you are using, consult Reading #24 or the general instructions on Rune Layouts in the Quick Reference Guide.

ACCESS POINTS

Runeless Readings: 4, 5, 6, 7, 10, 11, 12, 13, 20, 21, 22, 23

Make Runes: Reading #1 (How To); Extra, Extra Credit sections

Step-by-Step Encounter with Runes: Start at Reading #1

Go It Alone: Start at Reading #24

Choose a Question: Consult the Contents or Index

Complete Instructions: Reading #24

Notes on Layouts: Quick Reference Guide

Maximum Value: Appendix: How to Get Your Money's Worth

The Readings

Reading #1

IS THIS MY LUCKY DAY?
(Yes/no, tell me so)

In this Reading, you'll identify your "lucky charm" for today by simply choosing a letter of the alphabet . . . either an authentic ancient Runic character or—if you prefer—a modern English letter. In addition to getting your good-luck charm, you can also use this Reading to answer any yes/no question of your choosing.

ᚠ ᚠ ᚠ

RUNE TOOLS

In this Reading, we will be using the 24 oldest Runes known . . . the Runes that are as old as Europe. No wonder so many of them resemble the English letters passed down to us:

A	ᚠ	G	ᚷ	N	ᚾ	U	ᚢ
B	ᛒ	H	ᚺ	O	ᛟ	V	ᚹ
C	ᚲ	I	ᛁ	P	ᛈ	W	ᚹ
D	ᛞ	J	ᛃ	Q	ᚲ	X	*
Ê	ᛇ	K	ᚲ	R	ᚱ	Y	ᛃ
E	ᛗ	L	ᛚ	S	ᛋ	Z	ᛉ
F	ᚠ	M	ᛗ	T	ᛏ	Th	ᚦ
						-ing	ᛜ

☐ = The Blank Rune

* There is no Rune that makes the same sound as our letter X. In this book alphabet tile users will be using X as the Rune **-ing.**

3

But if you'd rather use your familiar ABC's, I'm sure the Ancestors won't mind one iota. Your Readings will work just the same and equally as well as the Runes they first invented.

HOW TO

1 First, you'll need a set of Runes.

To use "real" Runes. Either use the ones you already own, buy some from your favorite bookstore, or make some—which is really the most fun.

How to make notepad Runes. For a quick-and-dirty set of Runes—or to make Runes on the fly—all you need (really) is a pad of scratch paper. Tear off 25 sheets. Write one Rune onto one side of each sheet, leaving one sheet blank. Fold each square in half. Put them in a hat, and you're ready to begin. Your set of Runes will look like this:

To use alphabet tiles. A good alternative to Runes is the English-letter alphabet tiles from your Scrabble® board game. There are just three tricks . . .

- You'll need one each of the letter titles Ⓐ through Ⓩ <u>plus</u> both blanks and an extra Ⓔ. Put the rest of the tiles back in the box.

- Use one of the blank tiles for ᚦ **(Th)**, by penciling "Th" or "ᚦ" on one side of it: Ⓣ or Ⓣ. Leave the other blank tile, blank

- Next, pencil a triangle (or shape of your choice) above one of the letter *E*'s, Ⓔ. (This will show you which of the *E*'s in your set stands for short and silent *E*.)

4

Here is what your set of alphabet tiles will look like:

Ⓐ   Ⓑ   Ⓒ   Ⓓ   Ⓔ   Ⓔ́

Ⓕ   Ⓖ   Ⓗ   Ⓘ   Ⓙ   Ⓚ

Ⓛ   Ⓜ   Ⓝ   Ⓞ   Ⓟ   Ⓠ

Ⓡ   Ⓢ   Ⓣ   Ⓤ   Ⓥ   Ⓦ

Ⓧ   Ⓨ   Ⓩ   ⓣⱨ   ▢

Once you've got your set of Runes, you're ready to roll.

② To conduct this Reading, mix up your Runes while you think of your question. Ask: **What kind of luck will I have tomorrow?** in this venture? with my money? in my love life? **How lucky am I? Will my luck hold out?** in work, love, money, power . . . you name it, whatever you want to ask.

There is no right or wrong way to "mix up" your Runes, just "shuffle" them over in your hands or jumble them up in your Rune bag.

③ Now reach into your Runes and draw one out. Turn it over so you can see it. Look at it. And look it up in the answers that follow.

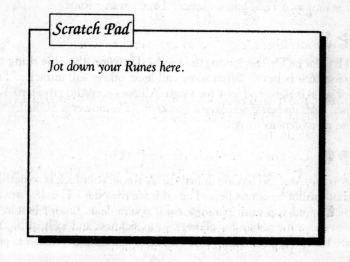

Scratch Pad

Jot down your Runes here.

THE ANSWERS

The answers appear in the traditional order of the Runes:

F U Th A R K G W H N I Y Ê P Z S T B E M L X O D

ᚠ ᚢ ᚦ ᚨ ᚱ ᚲ ᚷ ᚹ ᚺ ᚾ ᛁ ᛇ ᛃ ᛈ ᛉ ᛊ ᛏ ᛒ ᛖ ᛗ ᛚ ᛜ ᛟ ᛞ

☐ The Blank Rune appears last.   K=C & Q;   W=V;   Y=J

ᚠ Ⓕ

F is for **F**ortune. So having drawn the **F**-Rune, you are most fortunate, my friend . . . at life in general, but mostly at the things that
money buys. The future holds out hope for property deals under
favorable terms. *Your luck holds up best if you keep your fingers
crossed. The answer is YES, you strike it rich.*

ᚢ Ⓤ

U is for l**U**ck. So having drawn the **U**-Rune, you're just about as
lucky a son of a buck as ever crossed the turnpike in a fog. Things
go wrong for others, but not for you . . . not now . . . and not in general. Tread gently, my friend. They say that Lady Luck can change
her mind. *Your luck holds up best if you remember to knock on wood.
The answer is YES, take a chance. Draw another Rune.*

ᚦ Ⓣⓗ

Th is for fai**Th**. So having drawn the **Th**-Rune, the only thing you
must do is believe. What some call luck, others call miracles. Pray
for what is right and look for a sign. All goes according to Plan. *Your
luck holds up best if you keep a candle lit. The answer is SURELY . . .
but in mysterious ways.*

ᚨ Ⓐ

A is for f**A**te. So having drawn the **A**-Rune, your luck is something
that cannot be controlled. The odds are the odds. The dice are the
dice. And you must play the cards you're dealt . . . for better, for
worse . . . for richer, for poorer . . . in sickness and in health. You
are lucky at persevering. *Your luck holds up best if you try not to press*

it. The answer is DEFINITELY, if you work with all you've got to make it happen.

ᚱ Ⓡ

R is for **Reality.** So having drawn the R-Rune, the luck you see is what you get. Look on the bright side and all will connect. Look on the dark, and everything fragments. There is a reason for what is happening! See the good . . . even in the bad. *Your luck holds up best if you don't let the going get you down. The answer is* comme ci comme ça—MAYBE, MAYBE NOT—*it's all in the eye of the beholder, after all.*

ᚲ Ⓒ Ⓚ Ⓠ

C is for **Course.** **K** is for **Karma.** And **Q** is for **Quest.** So having drawn the C/K/Q-Rune, you are thrice lucky . . . especially when it comes to reaching the right conclusions and making the right decisions. Don't worry! There is a light at the end of this tunnel. Or is that a light going off in your head? *Your luck will hold up best if you go where the inspiration leads. The answer is MOST ASSUREDLY, as long as you follow the signs.*

ᚷ Ⓖ

G is for **Gifts.** So having drawn the G-Rune, you are lucky at things that take advantage of your natural talents and your native gifts. Live up to your full potential, and all the other pieces will fall into place. You are not so much lucky as blessed. And you can thank your lucky stars for this. *Your luck holds up best if you keep doing what you do best. The answer is YES, give it your best.*

ᚠ Ⓥ Ⓦ

W is for **Wonder.** **V** is for mar**V**elous. So having drawn the V/W-Rune, it would seem as if wonders never cease. Whatever brings you this time to the top of the wheel, you're riding high. You have the luck of the draw. You're on a winning streak. *Your luck holds up best if you play the odds. The answer is YOU BET . . . and you better believe it.*

H Ⓗ

H is for **Hail**. So having drawn the H-Rune, you're in for a little nasty weather. But not to fear. The rains that fall from these dark skies eventually will run off . . . and be forgotten. Lucky you learn your lessons the first time, even if they come hard and fast. *Your luck holds out best if you take no chances. The answer is NO WAY, my friend, not now. But try again later.*

✦ Ⓝ

N is for **Need**. So having drawn the N-Rune, your luck is about to turn . . . but not quite yet. First, there is a test to pass. And it will take strength and endurance. Lucky you have one heck of an indomitable human spirit working for you. *Your luck holds out best if you let it run its course. The answer is NO, NO, a thousand times NO. But don't let it get to you. Things can, do, and always will change.*

I Ⓘ

I is for **Ice**. So having drawn the I-Rune, your luck is a little slippery when wet. But things can go either way right now. Avenues are as likely to close as they are to open up to you. Watch your step! Plan your moves carefully, and you will be lucky at gliding by. *Your luck holds up best if you test it once or twice. The answer is WHO KNOWS? Go ahead, give it a try.*

◇ Ⓨ Ⓙ

Y is for **Year**. **J** is for **January**. **J** is for **June**. So having drawn the Y/J-Rune, it is clear your luck pans out in time. It is only by starting things that we stand the chance of completing them. You are lucky at being in the right place at the right time. *Your luck holds out best if you keep lots of irons in the fire. The answer is YES, and you deserve it.*

♪ Ⓔ [short and silent E]

Ê is for **hElp**. So having drawn the Ê-Rune, it is clear that luck will turn in your favor, even if at the last moment. But before you can receive help, you must seek it. You are lucky at finding a way out. *Your luck holds up best if you carry a little protection in your hip pocket. The answer is YES, but only by the skin of your teeth . . . and the hair of your chinny-chin-chin.*

P is for ho**P**e. So having drawn the **P**-Rune, your wishes are inclined to come true. So—as they say—be careful what you choose . . . and think twice before you throw your coin in the well. Nothing comes without its price. Lucky you know how to strike a good deal. *Your luck holds out best if you trust in it. The answer is YES, it's worth holding out hope for.*

Z is for re**SIS**tance. So having drawn the **Z**-Rune, you are lucky at hanging in there. Though the end may yet be bitter, you will have fought the good fight along the way. Hold on to that which matters most to you. Hold out. And be persistent. *Your luck holds up best if you display the sign of your belief. The answer is not written yet. There is no word. But in this case, NO NEWS IS GOOD NEWS.*

S is for **S**un. **S** is for **S**tars. So having drawn the **S**-Rune, things are looking up for you again. The pieces of the puzzle are falling into place. The lines are being drawn. And things are cycling back up in your favor. You are lucky at making a comeback. *Your luck holds up best if you roll with it. The answer is OF COURSE. There's no time like the present. All systems are go.*

T is for **T**riumph. So having drawn the **T**-Rune, it is your luck to get ahead quickly. Victory of this kind comes only suddenly . . . without time for a second thought. Lucky you are quick on your feet and fast on the draw. *Your luck holds up best in an emergency. The answer is YES, you have what it takes.*

ᛒ ⑧

B is for **Birth**. **B** is for re**Birth**. So having drawn the **B**-Rune, this is a time of deliverance.   You are making a personal transformation . . . and a life-altering transition. A rite of passage may even be in store. A safe cocoon is forsaken. An outworn skin is shed. A new life awaits. You are lucky when it comes to making fresh starts. *Your luck holds out best if you try not to resist. The answer is YES—take a deep breath.*

ᛗ ⓔ

E is for f**Emale**. So having drawn the **E**-Rune, your luck is in the hands of a woman. Look deep within yourself to find the answers. Lady Luck is on your side, but you must be open to her subtle ways. Watch for the signs. *Your luck holds up best if you follow your instincts. The answer is, IT'S INTUITIVELY OBVIOUS. But you must discover it for yourself.*

ᛗ ⓜ

M is for **Male**. So having drawn the **M**-Rune, it is clear that your luck is in the hands of a man. Think with your head. But go with your gut. And in the end, you will get lucky—if you are not already. *Your luck holds up best if you wear your lucky Speedos. The answer is SOME GUYS HAVE ALL THE LUCK, and this time you score.*

ᛚ ⓛ

L is for **Love**. So having drawn the **L**-Rune, you are lucky at love. But oh, this is a poignant Rune to draw. For Love knows pain and anguish just as well as triumph and joy. That which tugs at the heart is sure to leave its mark on the flesh. *Your luck holds out best if you give it half a chance. The answer is YES . . . YES . . . YES.*

❈ ⓧ

-ing is for be**ING**. So having drawn the **ING**-Rune, you are lucky to be having this life experience . . . this pleasure and pain . . . this agony and ecstasy . . . this triumph and tragedy. *Your luck holds up best if you share it with someone who shares the same interests as yours. The answer is MAKE LOVE, NOT WAR.*

✖ ⓞ

O is for h**O**me. So having drawn the O-Rune, you are lucky to have found where you fit in and where you belong. This place is your home now. These people are your people. And—the truth to tell—you would have it no other way. It is as it is. *Your luck holds out best if you let it rub off on others. The answer is YES . . . now, always, and forever and ever.*

✖ ⓓ

D is for **D**estiny. So having drawn the D-Rune, you have come full circle, and your luck has flip-flopped . . . and flop-flipped. You are back to square one, but older and wiser this time around. What have you learned? *Your luck holds up best if you take it with a grain of salt. The answer is YES, give it one more try.*

▯

The Blank Rune is . . . a little **weird**! Having drawn it, it is clear your luck is about to change . . . but which way will it go? Everything is possible now . . . and yet nothing is happening yet. *Your luck holds up best if you take life for what it's worth. The answer is BEATS ME. You make the call.*

EXTRA CREDIT

To ask any yes/no question by "casting" your Runes. Think of your question while you mix up your Runes. Then pick up a handful of Runes and toss them on the floor. If the majority fall Rune-side up, the answer is YES. If the majority fall Rune-side down, the answer is NO. For further information, read the *italic* portions of this Reading's answers for all your Runes that land faceup.

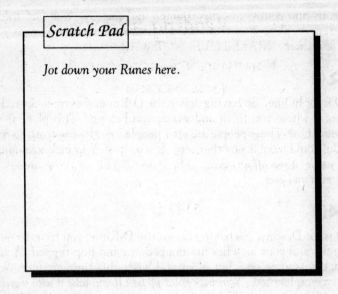

Scratch Pad

Jot down your Runes here.

EXTRA, EXTRA CREDIT!

To make a simple Yes/No Rune. Find yourself a flat, smooth skipping-type stone or wood chip and—with a permanent marker or a little paint (red is traditional)—mark one side YES (or YEA) and the other side NO (or NAY). To ask your question, clasp your Yes/No Rune between the palms of your hands, think of your question, and say, **Yes/no tell me so.** Throw your stone on the floor. The side that lands faceup is your answer. Instead of actually throwing your stone (those who live in glass houses shouldn't!), you can also toss it gently back and forth in your hands a few times. When you "feel" the answer has come, let the stone land in one hand. Read the sign.

Yea / **Nay** ,   **Yes** / **No**

Go on to the next Reading whenever you are ready to continue.

Reading #2

WHAT WILL TOMORROW BRING?
(Send me a sign)

In this Reading, you'll use your Runes to get a 24-hour forecast for the day that lies ahead. You can also use it to assess the outcome for just about anything—from today's love affair to tomorrow's real estate deal.

ᚢ ᚢ ᚢ

RUNE TOOLS

We will continue to work with the 24 traditional European Runes we used in Reading #1. In traditional Runic order, they are . . .

ᚠ	F	ᚷ	G	ᛃ	Ê	ᛗ	E
ᚢ	U	ᚹ	V/W	ᛈ	P	ᛖ	M
ᚦ	Th	ᚺ	H	ᛉ	Z	ᛚ	L
ᚨ	A	ᚾ	N	ᛊ	S	ᛝ	-ing (X)
ᚱ	R	ᛁ	I	ᛏ	T	ᛟ	O
ᚲ	C/K/Q	ᛇ	Y/J	ᛒ	B	ᛞ	D

In recent years, a Blank Rune has been added at the end: **☐** So we shall use it, too.

13

HOW TO

1   To conduct this Reading, do the same thing you did in Reading #1. Just think of your question: **What will tomorrow bring?** in general? with regard to my love life? for my money? in my career? **How will everything turn out?** for the company? the country? the two of us? **What will I have at the end of the day?**

2   Now, with your question in mind, shake up your Runes (or alphabet tiles). Reach into your Rune bag, feel around for the one that wants to be drawn, and take it out of the bag.

3   Look up your Rune in the Answers, and read what *Runes in Ten Minutes* has to say.

Scratch Pad

Jot down your Runes here.

THE ANSWERS

The answers appear in the traditional order of the Runes:

F U Th A R K G W H N I Y Ê P Z S T B E M L X O D

ᚠ ᚢ ᚦ ᚨ ᚱ ᚲ ᚷ ᚹ ᚺ ᚾ ᛁ ᛃ ᛇ ᛈ ᛉ ᛊ ᛏ ᛒ ᛖ ᛗ ᛚ ᛜ ᛟ ᛞ

▢ The Blank Rune appears last. K=C & Q; W=V; Y=J

14

F Ⓕ

Tomorrow brings **F**ortune, my friend . . . good fortune and even a certain amount of fame. Regrettably, these two and wealth do not always go hand in hand. But you will have plenty to be envied of in this life. And at the end of the day, you will have many things to add up on your calculator.

U Ⓤ

Tomorrow brings good l**U**ck, my friend. So get out there and break a leg . . . or at least a wishbone. What's down, goes up. What's up, comes down. And the magic wheel goes round and round. By the end of the day, you'll have something to thank your lucky stars about.

Þ Ⓣ̲ₕ

Tomorrow brings you fai**Th**, my friend . . . and devotion. Everything goes according to Plan. So say a prayer and sleep well, knowing that the morning follows midnight. When everything else is done—and all is spoken—you'll have a shoulder to lean on at the end of the day.

Ꮭ Ⓐ

Tomorrow brings f**A**te, my friend . . . so I guess you might say it's in the cards. It's in the bag. And there's nothing you can do now but wait for the hours to pass. Your own past catches up to you, and all the pieces fall in place. By the end of the day you will know what it all adds up to . . . even if you don't know why.

R Ⓡ

Tomorrow brings a **R**eality check . . . and a certain restlessness some call the wanderlust. There are hard questions to be asked and answered—but mostly of, and by, yourself. Where have you come from? Where does it all lead? By sunset you shall have journeyed far indeed.

< Ⓒ Ⓚ Ⓠ

Tomorrow brings the whitening sky of a new day . . . and a fresh outlook on an old world. It would seem as if your Course is set now, and your Quest over. Leave the rest to kismet . . . and to Karma. By the end of the day, you will see the light.

✕ Ⓖ

Tomorrow brings Gifts . . . both given and received, in an exchange of favors, if not also feelings, sentiments, and words. The senses and emotions mix. You may even feel tingles. Don't forget to say the magic words. At the end of the day, you'll feel on top of the world.

Ᵽ Ⓥ Ⓦ

Tomorrow brings a little bundle of joy . . . and the childlike sense of Wonder that brings magic to the world. Can this really be happening? Quick, pinch yourself! Then treasure the moment that passes too fast. At the end of the day, you'll wish you had it all to do over again.

Ⲯ Ⓗ

Tomorrow brings Hail . . . wind and rain . . . flash floods . . . high tides . . . and fallen limbs. There are but two routes to take. What say ye? Ride out the storm . . . or move to safer ground? By the end of the day, the decision will be made . . . whether it is right, or whether it is wrong.

✚ Ⓝ

Tomorrow brings Need . . . want . . . desire . . . yearning. You crave the taste of fruit out of season . . . long for a cigarette on the plane . . . pine for the love you cannot have. Misery, they say, loves company, but has few friends. By the end of the day, you will be pulling yourself back together again.

❘ Ⓘ

Tomorrow brings Ice . . . snow . . . freezing rain . . . and frozen patches on the bridges and overpasses. Things are closing in around you and opening up at the same time. Those with skates can cross the river now. All others must stay where they are. By the end of the day, you will know whether the forecasters were right.

◇ Ⓨ Ⓙ

Tomorrow brings the end of a **Y**ear . . . a change in the seasons . . . and the start of a new cycle. The days have come and gone. The Full Moon rises, revealing all that is left now to glean from another growing season. Take up what is yours. Reap what you have sown. By the end of the day, you will receive your just reward.

♩ Ⓔ

Tomorrow brings h**E**lp. And it's about time that help came! But you will need to defend yourself in the process . . . show your faith . . . put up a good front . . . keep a stiff upper lip . . . and maybe even carry a lucky charm. By the end of the day, you shall have averted danger.

Ⓚ Ⓟ

Tomorrow brings ho**P**e . . . and yours is springing eternal. It's a day for pursuing dreams, wishes, and ambitions—even if they are sky-high. You might have to risk something in order to win something. But at the end of the day, you will know whether your hunch paid off this time.

Ⓨ Ⓩ

Tomorrow brings re**SIS**tance . . . persistence . . . and endurance in response to a real or perceived threat. Wear the signs of your faith upon your breast. Make the sign of the cross. Say a prayer. By the end of the day, you will have proved that the strength of your own beliefs will see you through.

Ⓢ Ⓢ

Tomorrow brings **S**unrise, morning **S**tar . . . and a brand new day. The light in your life that was hidden in darkness suddenly returns.

The winter is over. The summer has come. This is your window of opportunity . . . to shine. By the end of the day, you will have no regrets, save that the day is done.

↑ Ⓣ

Tomorrow brings **T**riumph . . . and a sudden switching of the odds to your favor. The dart hits the bull's-eye. And good for you! At last you earn the credit that's long overdue. Stand tall. Enjoy your moment of glory. By the end of the day, you will be lifted up on somebody's shoulders.

ᛒ Ⓑ

Tomorrow brings **B**irth . . . and re**B**irth. And this, my friend, is that pregnant moment on the eve of change. What was, now passes away for good. A new life starts . . . and everything is possible again. By the end of the day, you'll feel like a whole new person.

ᛗ Ⓔ

Tomorrow favors the f**E**male in you . . . and the women in your life. It's a good day to call your mother, go out with the girls, or spend time as a family. Share what you've been thinking. Tell how you've been feeling. By the end of the day, your spirits will have improved immensely.

ᛗ Ⓜ

Tomorrow favors men . . . the men in your life . . . good buddies . . . best friends . . . and **M**ale activities of all kinds. This is a time for bonding and binding. A partnership deal is sealed with a hand-shake, if not also a kiss. By the end of the day, you will have come to a mutual agreement.

ᚱ Ⓛ

Tomorrow, my friend, brings **L**ove and comfort . . . from family and friends, especially . . . but not excluding lovers. The heart hungers for the company of others from the same clan. Blood relatives, blood brothers, and bosom buddies are involved. By the end of the day, you'll feel as if you belong to each other.

✖ ⊠

Tomorrow favors be**ING** who you are . . . especially in bed. Sleep in. Take a nap. Or use your imagination. The Universe is one big act of creation. And all that it asks of you now is that you be creative. By the end of the day, you will have come close to nirvana.

✖ ⊙

Tomorrow favors things at h**O**me. It's a good day for puttering around . . . cleaning, polishing, mowing, sweeping—but all in its own good time. You might even want to sleep in. What does it cost you if something doesn't get checked off the list? By the end of the day, you'll have made plenty of progress.

▷◁ ⊙

Tomorrow brings **D**estiny, my friend . . . and what a difference a day makes! One stage is wrapped up now, and it's time for a new era to begin. A letter arrives in the mail, or the phone rings. And by the end of the day, your own actions will have swayed the outcome and altered your fate.

◻

Tomorrow something **weird** will happen, but—not to fear—it's all in the cards. And by the end of the day, a lot of things will be explained.

EXTRA CREDIT

To receive a sign. You don't even have to ask a question to get valuable information from the Runes. Just clear your mind of idle thoughts as you mix them up. When you're feeling peaceful and mellow, say, **Give me a sign**, and fish out the first Rune you can get ahold of. Look it up in this Reading's Answer section. And if the shoe fits, don't be surprised.

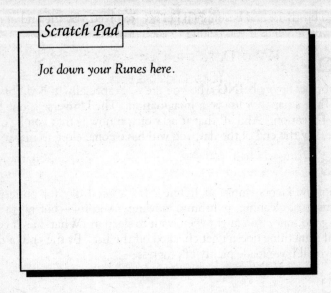

Scratch Pad

Jot down your Runes here.

EXTRA, EXTRA CREDIT!

How to make matchstick Runes. To make an authentic set of Runes in a hurry, <u>cut the heads off</u> of 25 large wooden kitchen matches (Ohio Blue Tips are great). With a red felt-tip pen or marker of your choice, inscribe one of the Runes on each match, leaving one whole matchstick blank. Think of your question (you can ask anything). Toss your Runesticks on the floor. Pick one from the heap. And look it up in the Quick Reference Guide's Master Answer section.

Matchstick Runes are great for those who want to start with a fresh set of Runes each time. For a truly authentic Runic experience, burn your Runes in an ashtray when your session is done.

Go on to the next Reading whenever you are ready to continue.

Reading #3

WHAT DOES THE PAST ADD UP TO?
(Show 'n' tell me)

In this Reading, you'll consult your Runes in order to learn what the past has to say about your future. By taking a quick look back, the Reading will help you glimpse the larger picture. What was it all about? Where did it all lead? And where should you go from here?

ᚠᚠᚠ

RUNE TOOLS

The Runes you are using are known as the "Elder Futhark." "Elder," because they are the oldest set of Runes known. "Futhark," because that's the meaningless word formed by the first six letters of these Runic ABC's. Repeat after me. . . .

ᚠ ᚢ ᚦ ᚨ ᚱ ᚲ

F U Th A R K

The Runes of the Elder Futhark are the same Runes we used in Readings #1 and #2. Now you know an easy way to recall how their sequence starts. Just remember, the magic word is: **F U Th A R K.**

HOW TO

To use your Runes or alphabet tiles to conduct this Reading, just . . .

1 Think of your question: **What does my past add up to?** in love? at work? with money? **What is the lesson of my life experience?** my past loves? past homes? past jobs?

2 With your question in mind, mix up your Runes. Reach

into your bag and draw out the one that calls your name.

3　Look up your Rune in this Reading's Answer section.

Scratch Pad

Jot down your Runes here.

THE ANSWERS

The answers appear in the traditional order of the Runes:

F U Th A R K G W H N I Y Ê P Z S T B E M L X O D

ᚠ ᚢ ᚦ ᚨ ᚱ ᚲ ᚷ ᚹ ᚺ ᚾ ᛁ ᛇ ᛃ ᛈ ᛉ ᛊ ᛏ ᛒ ᛖ ᛗ ᛚ ᛜ ᛟ ᛞ

☐ The Blank Rune appears last.　K=C & Q; W=V; Y=J

ᚠ Ⓕ

You have been **F**ortunate, my friend. For things have added up quite well for you, like trophies on a hunter's wall. And you have been blessed—oh, let me count the many ways and hows and wheres and whyfors. Yet . . . *You have been trying to learn that every-*

thing is relative. The best advice is, take stock, especially of the things that can be numbered only by the heart.

ᚢ Ⓤ

You have been lUcky in the past . . . you lucky duck! For things have not just gone your way, they have gone out of their way to go yours. And just when you needed it most, miracles occurred. A path through the wilderness has been cleared for you. *You have been trying to learn that luck counts, too, even if it's dumb. The best advice is, don't muck with a winning streak.*

ᚦ Ⓣₕ

You have been faiThful in the past . . . true to The Word, perhaps. Most certainly true to <u>your</u> words . . . a martyr to the cause, if not also a saint in your deeds. Your life is a testament to your beliefs. *You have been trying to learn that faith untested is just lip service. The best advice is, say your prayers but be prepared to fight for your religion.*

ᚨ Ⓐ

Your past was simply fAted. It just had to be that way. And now that all is said and done, it could have gone no better . . . and you come out no worse for wear. So here we are, my friend, at last together. What shall we do with this moment when we might change things forever? *You have been trying to overcome your past. The best advice is, move on. But first, make your wish and draw another Rune.*

ᚱ Ⓡ

Your past adds up to the Real thing . . . and suddenly you find yourself staring Reality in the face. So this is what it was all about. And this is what your future used to be. If you had known, would you have headed in another direction? As always, the question is, where do you go from here? *You have been trying to learn how to choose. The best advice is, ask. Cast your Runes again.*

< Ⓒ Ⓚ Ⓠ

Your past adds up to an endless **Q**uest . . . a sure **C**ourse . . . and an eternal play of **K**armic force. Do you think it could possibly have been so fickle a thing as luck to have brought you to this spot? A light goes off in your head. *You have been trying to learn that the past is only part of your mission. The best advice is, put it behind you now . . . set your sights anew, and full steam ahead.*

✕ Ⓖ

The past has given you, lo, these many **G**ifts: the ones you were born with . . . the ones you acquired, the ones you gave up in exchange, and the ones you gave from the heart. These tell the whole story of everything until now . . . the credits and debits, the pros and the cons, the givings and takings, and the goings back and forth. *You have been trying to learn that it truly is the thought that counts. The best advice is, send roses.*

⊳ Ⓥ Ⓦ

Your past has had its joyous, **W**ondrous moments. You have known your share of happiness . . . ecstasy . . . even wild-eyed wonder. And it is not just the way things were . . . for the mark the past has left on you is as indelible as laugh lines. *You have been trying to learn that, despite its serious moments, life is pretty funny. The best advice is, hold on to the night.*

Ⓗ Ⓗ

Your past has had its **H**ail and hardships, my friend. And you have known your share of troubles . . . some small and some the size of golf balls. Into each life—or so they say—a little rain (and hail!) befalls us. The Fickle Finger of Fate has pointed in your general direction, yet you have survived. *You have been trying to learn what it means to overcome. The best advice is, breathe deeply and gather your courage to go on.*

✝ Ⓝ

In the past you have **N**eeded many things . . . and known your share of want—perhaps even suffered a tragedy or two. At the very least, you've been down on your luck. But it's all relative, of course. In the end—as they say—you'll be stronger for it. *You've been trying to learn the facts of life . . . the hard way. The best advice is, observe the phases of the moon, and see for yourself how everything comes back around.*

I ⓘ

In the past you've known your share of snow and wind and **I**ce. Perhaps you were even a little icy yourself . . . constricted . . . restricted . . . frozen and fettered—but oh, so smooth to the touch. What was the hunger yearning at your center? What was the fire within? *You have been trying to learn how to heed your call. The best advice is, break loose when you can, wait when you must.*

❖ ⓨ ⓙ

The past **Y**ear or so has been a turning point for you. And now that you stand at the end of a full cycle looking back, you can clearly see how it all turns out. What did these seeds of the past yield in the end? What have you gleaned from this experience? What can you harvest? *You have been trying to learn to see a pattern in the larger scheme of things. The best advice is, quickly gather as much as you can of all that remains.*

♩ ⬆

In the past, you were in need of h**E**lp, my friend. But—lo and behold—help came at last, did it not? And you saw your way clear . . . even from potential ruin and disaster. What was your secret— positive thinking? Prayer? A little magic? Or was it plain old luck? *You have been trying to learn how to trust. The best advice is, don't forget to wear your lucky socks.*

↖ ⓟ

In the past you have ho**P**ed . . . perhaps against all odds . . . that the impossible would happen. You have taken your share of chances. You have put your money on the line . . . perhaps even risked all. At least no one can say you didn't play the cards you were dealt. *You* *have been trying to learn how to influence the luck of the draw. The best advice is, double or nothing, pal.*

Ψ Ⓩ

In the past you have known reSIStance, and resilience. You have worried your fair share. You have even feared the unknown. But for the most part you have warded off danger. All in all, you have had your health—though you have worried your share about losing it. *You have been trying to learn that the days are counted as well as numbered. The best advice is, use it or lose it.*

⟨ Ⓢ

In the past you have known **S**unshine . . . and **S**tarlight. You have counted up days you wished would last and the nights you did not want to pass. So days have added up to weeks, and weeks to moons, and moons to years. And now another cycle starts. *You have been trying to learn that everything old becomes new again. The best advice is, watch for a comet, count shooting stars, wish upon a Crescent Moon, and draw another Rune.*

↑ Ⓣ

In the past you have known moments of **T**riumph . . . been held up on the shoulders of others . . . rode in the lead car . . . stood on the pedestal . . . and done your share of victory dances down the line. But oh, how fleeting are the moments of glory—as brief as youth itself. Yet they leave this lasting mark, and this constant pining for more. *You have been trying to learn what it means to be a hero. The best advice is, keep giving it your best shot.*

Ｂ Ⓑ

In the past you gave **B**irth (or was it you who was re**B**orn?).The infant struggles at first, then learns to crawl, and then to stand. You too have finally pulled yourself up on your own two feet—and in so doing, have walked the longest mile. *You have been trying to learn that life is a series of endings and fresh starts . . . landmarks, crossroads,* *and turning points. The best advice is, take a deep breath and start all over again.*

M Ⓔ

In the past there was a fEmale in your life . . . a mother, lover, sister, friend, or spouse. At any rate there was a strong womanly influence—or the woman in you expressed herself. But what shall you do with this intuitive advice? How shall you react to your fate? And how shall you feel your way to your destiny? *You have been trying to learn how to open up. The best advice is, listen to the voices that give you good advice.*

⋈ Ⓜ

In the past there was a **Male** in your life . . . a brother, father, mentor, lover, friend, or spouse. At the very least, a strong manly influence dominated you. Or the man in you expressed himself in a series of overt acts and outward accomplishments. In some respects, the whole experience has "made a man" of you. *You have been trying to learn how to make things happen. The best advice is, use plenty of elbow grease.*

ᚱ Ⓛ

In the past you have known **Love** of one sort or another (for love knows many names, kinds, and varieties). You have run both gauntlet and gambit. You have ranged from hot to cold. But of the feelings that brother feels for brother and the mother for her child, there is no doubt in your heart. *You have been trying to learn that blood is thicker than water. The best advice is, open up.*

✸ Ⓧ

In the past you have encountered your sexual be**ING** . . . the force that drives you to do as you do, to say what you say, and to be who you are. The good Lord has done well to never make the same snowflake twice. And of diversity there is no end in this Great Universe of ours. *You have been trying to learn how to express yourself. The best advice is, turn the lights down low.*

✠ ⍥

In the past you have felt at h**O**me . . . with your life, with your world, with the people about you, and—if you were lucky—even with yourself. For though you have journeyed far, this is the place to which you return . . . this is the center of your Universe. *You have been trying to learn that everything connects to everything else. The best advice is, follow the heartstrings that tug.*

⋈ ⍥

In the past you have had a glimpse of **D**estiny . . . and you have felt a sense of purpose. Your past is like a continuous loop that twists round and round on itself in an endless, repetitive pattern. If you would know the future, my friend, it is written plainly on your past. *You have been trying to learn, not how to break the pattern, but how to work with it. The best advice is, accept rather than resist . . . work with, rather than against.*

⍥

In the past it's been **weird** that you have not been able to find the words to express your feelings or the data that supports your conclusions. The Universe is full of darkness marked by patches of intermittent light. But it takes both to hold it all together. *You have been trying to learn how you fit into the scheme of things. The best advice is, pay attention to your dreams.*

EXTRA CREDIT

For a quick piece of advice. To ask about any matter that concerns you, mix up your Runes while you think of your question: **What have I been trying to learn? What should I do about _____?** Or, simply, with your issue in mind, say, **Show and tell me.** Draw out as many Runes as come into your hand at once. Or to cast your Runes, take a handful and throw them on the floor. Read for those that land Rune-side up. Consult the *italic* portion of this Reading's answers.

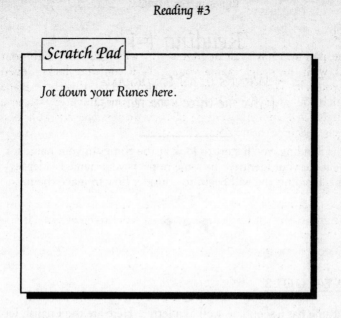

Scratch Pad

Jot down your Runes here.

EXTRA, EXTRA CREDIT!

To conduct a past, present, and future Reading. Think of the matter that concerns you while you mix up your Runes. Ask your question: **How should I proceed with regard to _____?** Reach into your Runes and draw out three.

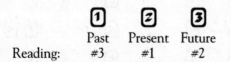

	Past	**Present**	**Future**
Reading:	#3	#1	#2

The first Rune you draw represents the past. Look it up in the answers here in Reading #3. The second Rune you draw represents the present. Look it up in the answers to Reading #1. The third Rune represents the future. Look it up in the answers to Reading #2.

Go on to the next Reading whenever you are ready to continue.

Reading #4

WHAT'S IN A MONOGRAM?
(Give me three good reasons)

———

In this Reading, you'll start to look at the Runes in your name for clues about your identity. In some respects your name is a legacy. In this Reading you will begin to consider how to make the most of yours.

ᚠ ᚠ ᚠ

RUNE TOOLS

Each Rune has a sound, as well as a letter. Here are the English letters, along with the Runes that sound like them:

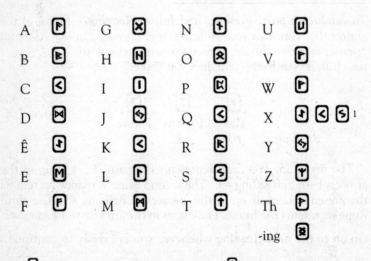

[1] Use ᚷ, if the *x* actually makes a *g* sound. Use ᛉ, if the *x* actually makes a *z* sound.

HOW TO

To find out what your initials have to say about you . . .

1   Jot down your first, middle, and last initials on the Scratch Pad. Also jot down the initials of others you are interested in asking about.

> ### Scratch Pad
>
> *Jot down your initials here.*

2   Now look up your initials in the chart in this Reading's Tools section. Write the corresponding Runes on the Scratch Pad. There are just three tricks. . . .

■   If any of your initials is an *E*, you'll have to decide between the two Runes that have an *E* sound: *E* as in Ethan (**M**) or *Ê* as in Edward (**↑**).

■   If any of your names begins with the letters *Th*, use the **Th**-Rune (**Þ**) in the appropriate place.

■   If you lack, say, a middle name, use the blank Rune (**□**). Or if *ing* appears anywhere in your name, use the **ING**-Rune (**❈**).

In the rare event that one of your initials is an X, there is no equivalent-sounding Rune. So you'll have to use a Rune that sounds the same. Use the **Z**-Rune for Xavier (ᛉ). Use the **E**-, **K**-, and **S**-Runes for Malcolm's X (ᛖ ᚲ ᛋ). Or you may find that K (ᚲ) or G (ᚷ) does the trick for you.

③   Look up your Runes in this Reading's Answer section. Read the whole answer for each of your initials, but for your first initial, focus on the part of the answer called "*In the first place.*" For your middle initial, focus on "*In the second place.*" And for your last name, focus on "*In the third place,*" but also read the text for "*In all cases.*"

THE ANSWERS

The answers appear in the traditional order of the Runes:

F U Th A R K G W H N I Y Ê P Z S T B E M L X O D

ᚠ ᚢ ᚦ ᚨ ᚱ ᚲ ᚷ ᚹ ᚺ ᚾ ᛁ ᛃ ᛇ ᛈ ᛉ ᛋ ᛏ ᛒ ᛖ ᛗ ᛚ ᛝ ᛟ ᛞ

ᛟ **The Blank Rune appears last.   K=C & Q; W=V; Y=J**

ᚠ Ⓕ

There is **F**ortune in your name. And fortunate, you shall be . . . in one way or another. For you desire the things that can be counted up, as well as counted upon . . . numbered, as well as named.

①   *In the first place* you are fortunate in being able to draw to yourself the things that mark you as affluent. Take stock of your lifestyle and say thanks.

②   *In the second place* you are fortunate in the ideas that possess you. They tend to be right on the money. You have a good head on your neck. Use it.

③   *In the third place* you are fortunate in the possessions that have been handed down to you. Guard your inheritance. Protect your legacy. Collect your birthright.

In all cases bigger is not necessarily better. But as long as there is breath within you, you shall aspire for more. Take a deep one, and count to three.

∪ ⓤ

There is lUck in your name. And lucky you are, my friend. For things go your way in general, and the bad passes quickly. You want the dice to roll 7's and 11's. You want the wheel of chance to hold still while you ride out the winning streak. And good luck—it seems—watches over you like an angel.

❶ *In the first place* you are lucky about being in the right lane at the right time. All you have to do is drive within the lines, and you will get there.

❷ *In the second place* you are lucky in sensing when the moment has come to pull out into the passing lane. So don't play chicken.

❸ *In the third place* you are lucky in the cards you have been dealt. Thank the folks for their great genes. And be sure to count the family luck among your hand-me-downs.

In all cases your life is always sweeter when you take a risk. So live on the verge if you must, but never on the edge. Hold the cruise control to 62.

ᚦ ⓣⓗ

There is faiTh written within your name. So what choice do you have but to believe? You desire to know The Answer. Seek and ye shall find, I guess—but what more do you wish to learn than what your heart already knows? You can relate to the things that stir the soul.

❶ *In the first place* you are faithful to the ones who matter to you and to the ones whom you matter to. Keep your pledge to one another.

❷ *In the second place* you are faithful to the Word within you. Renew your sacred vows at least once a week.

❸ *In the third place* you are faithful to the blood relations. Preserve the ways of your own people as well as their DNA.

In all cases your faith will sustain you. *Om Mani Padme Hum. Shalom.* Amen.

ᚠ Ⓐ

Your name has fAte written upon it. And in so many words, you are destined to achieve much . . . over this and many lifetimes. They say our past comes round to save us or back to haunt us, and that the scales even out over time. Avoid making the same mistakes twice. Try to learn your lessons the first time.

① *In the first place* your flesh is willing. Take your fate in your own two hands. It is never too late to change, set goals, or make amends.

② *In the second place* your spirit is willing. If at first you don't succeed, you know what to do. But just in case you've forgotten the punch line, keep plugging.

③ *In the third place* your blood is not just thick, it's willing. Work with the strengths and weaknesses you have inherited. You can turn even the family curse into a cure.

In all cases though your life may be a familiar situation, only you can write its surprise ending. Live and learn, my friend. Learn and live.

ᚱ Ⓡ

Your name has Reality written all over it. So ranting, raving, railing against the odds, you see it all for what it is . . . is not . . . and yet could be. You have no choice but to follow your own dream no matter what seems real or unreal to others . . . and no matter how far they think it's leading you astray.

① *In the first place* you know yourself pretty well, or will by the time you finish this journey. Keep testing. Keep proving what you need to prove.

② *In the second place* you have a vision of how things ought to be. Picture it. See it. Imagine it as coming true. Then work to bring that vision into reality.

③ *In the third place* you come from a long line of seekers and searchers. If there's no one in your immediate clan who's quite the right role model, pay a visit to your long-lost cousins.

In all cases you follow in the footsteps of those who have walked your way before. Seek guidance from the elders. But trust only that which feels true to you.

◀ Ⓒ Ⓚ Ⓠ

Your name is full of light. And with it comes your sense of **K**armic purpose. You are a person with a mission to achieve, a plan to fulfill, and a goal to reach. Follow your life **C**ourse. Stay true to your eternal **Q**uest. Home in on the light that guides you. Let the Source do the rest.

1 *In the first place* you are an energetic person. Put all of those amperes and kilowatts to work in your life. Shed your own light.

2 *In the second place* you are an inspired person. Incubate your random thoughts. Watch and wait for the revelations to come with sudden clarity.

3 *In the third place* you hail from a long line of people who have seen a great deal. Add your insights to the collective experience.

In all cases you shine with the light of your own being. Some heavenly lights burn red. Some are yellow . . . some, orange. Some even are blue. Be the color you were meant to be. Shine true.

✖ Ⓖ

Your name is full of **G**ifts . . . talents, abilities, propensities, skills, crafts . . . indeed, your name itself is a gift (for better or worse). As with anything you're given, all these things are yours to make the most of. Use them as you will. Combine them into something new that you give back.

1 *In the first place* there are many things you can choose to do with your time. Get maintenance and subsistence out of the way. Free up the hours for your creative works.

2 *In the second place* no one has to tell you how you ought to spend your time. Listen to that little voice in your head that knows best, as well as better. Do what it says.

3   *In the third place* you have the support of those who want to see you use your gifts. And they will help you all they can to make the most of yourself. But you must do the rest.

In all cases you have cause to delight. Unwrap your presents. Play with your toys. Open the doors in your head. Explore your inner sanctum.

▶ Ⓥ Ⓦ

There is **W**onder in your name. And so, you have no choice but to be inquisitive. It's a magical and joyous world to behold, my friend. And you are inclined to study it, appreciate it for what it is, and maybe even laugh at it for what it is not and can never be. You have the right (and healthy) outlook.

1   *In the first place* you have wide eyes—all the better to see with, my dear—as well as open ears. Look. Hear. See. Know. Take it all in . . . even the erogenous zones.

2   *In the second place* you have a receptive mind. Open yourself up to the possibilities. Try out different positions. Wear different clothes. Taste different things.

3   *In the third place* you come from a long line of people who agreed it was better to laugh at life than bemoan it. So if it tickles your funny bone, laugh. It's your best medicine.

In all cases go with a smile on your face. Have a blast on the way. And if the others can't take a joke . . . ah, kismet.

ᚺ Ⓗ

There is a bolt of thunder in your name . . . a flash of lightning . . . a little rain . . . and sudden **H**ail. Just like the weather map, you have your HIs and LOs, with intermittent periods of alternating calm and blowout. But what the heck, you wanted your life to be exciting, didn't you?

1   *In the first place* you like to see the fireworks on the Fourth of July as much as anybody else. Say ooooh! Say aaaaah! But don't let me catch *you* lobbing cherry bombs.

2   *In the second place* you can empathize with an episode of True Life Emergencies as well as the next citizen. But if you're going to go bungee-jumping, don't even think of suing the rope company.

3   *In the third place* you come from a people that not only knows how to get by, but has proved it can survive the thrill of the adventure. Follow in the footsteps. But wear the appropriate athletic gear.

In all cases you thrive on the right amount of stress. The storms that blow through your life also blow away. And it's a lucky thing your body's drip-dry.

✝ **N**

Need is written on the face of your name. But what of that? All who walk the earth are needy. And whatever your lot in life, there are always some who have it worse off. But with a Rune like this in your name, you not only want and need, you also burn with desire.

1   *In the first place* you yearn for a warm bed as well as a full belly. When there is no lean to eat, chew the fat. And if the house gets cold and damp, share the coverlet.

2   *In the second place* you cannot escape the endless urge that gnaws in you. Appease that which demands to be fed. Wet that which demands to be quenched. Put a lid on that which eats you out of house and home.

3   *In the third place* your family is living proof that even the wilderness can be beat. They got by on far less than you have. Use the tools they bequeathed you.

In all cases be sensitive to the needs of others. Nobody is alone here. Help out your family members. Rescue strangers. Accept a helping hand yourself. We're all going to pull through it all together.

❘ **I**

Your name has Ice in it . . . firm of resolve . . . and strong in its stillness. The way is smooth for you, but—careful now—it's also slick.

And what firms up also restricts. You want to lead a structured life, or else—poor child—you feel restricted by the rules. Conform or tough it out, I guess—the choice is yours.

1   *In the first place* you are firm in your beliefs and true in your convictions. Accept what you will. Decide what you can. Then do what you must.

2   *In the second place* you are good at self-restraint and self-control . . . but also self-indulgence. When in doubt, retreat into your shelter and make resolutions.

3   *In the third place* you come from a long line of those who kept their resolve in the face of all manner of adversity. If it snows on you, build an ice fort and crawl in.

In all cases you are molded by the conditions you endure. When times are tight, squeeze. But be ready to flow again, when things free up.

◇ ⟨ ◊

Time is operating in your name . . . the great cycle of the Year rolling round and round on itself, from start to finish, and from beginning to end. So, too, your life is like the unfolding of the seasons. You want the time to last. Yet you know that all things pass. There is a time to work and a time to rest.

1   *In the first place* you are good at making maximum use of your time. Get a head start on as many days as you can get the jump on. And burn the midnight oil for as many nights as you can function.

2   *In the second place* you are wise beyond your years. Draw from your own experience, as well as from the books, songs, and poems that have molded your thinking.

3   *In the third place* you can always learn a thing or two from the past. Put to use the information that's been handed down. Get yourself an almanac. And watch for the moon.

In all cases you are sure to make progress. From phase to phase, your life unfolds. Wax. Wane. And cycle back again. Work. Rest. And play.

♪ Ê

There is hElp in your name. So, in your life, help will always be standing by. Food, clothing, shelter, and medicine will come as needed. Enemies will have second thoughts. Even accidents will somehow avert you. And the money will always be enough.

① *In the first place* you are able to avoid trouble by watching out for it. So take care. Exert caution. And know when to panic. Worry has prevented more accidents than seat belts.

② *In the second place* you believe in powers greater than yourself. When in need, say a prayer. Summon the Saints and other intercessors. Or else invoke the Deity by dialing direct. (I hear they'll even accept collect.)

③ *In the third place* you come from a long line of folks who have done it all, seen it all, and come through it all many times before. Learn by example. Apply the family axioms and mottoes.

In all cases you are able to overcome the difficulties you face by practicing common sense. Rely on both the wit and wisdom of the ages. Take stock in the family sage.

◪ Ᵽ

There is hoPe in your name. And so—against all odds—you are sure to hope ever, and hope on. (Or is that hope on, hope ever?) Whatever. Each sunrise brings potential . . . each night, another chance. But you can't win if you don't play. And you can't play without taking a risk.

① *In the first place* you know a good hot dog when you smell it on the air . . . even if it is a little risky to eat anything that comes from green water. Take a calculated risk. Hold the sauerkraut. (But onions are lucky.)

② *In the second place* you have a feeling for when your luck is smiling on you. A roll is a roll. And they generally come eight to the package. Don't bite off more than you can chew at one time.

③ *In the third place* your kinfolk have always been gamblers, at least when it came to pursuing their dreams. But some did better than others. Adopt the winningest strategy of the bunch.

In all cases the American dream of lucking out is alive and well, and living in your heart. The answer to a prayer could be in that next scratch-and-win ticket. But just in case, you better keep your day job.

ᚊ Ⓩ

There is reSIStance in your name. So you have the power, my friend, to hold off disease, stand off oppressive forces, and ward off bad influences. Muster your full strength, and you stand a pretty good chance of doing all three. And it never hurts to leverage your faith.

① *In the first place* you have a body that doesn't need to be worshiped to do its job. Keep it in the best shape you can . . . by putting it to useful work. But don't forget who lent you those flat abdominals.

② *In the second place* you have a soul that also needs to be tended. Since it is the real source of your power, keep it on a high-fat diet of inspirational words. But don't forget it has a sweet tooth too.

③ *In the third place* you come from a long line of people who believed in what they were doing. Do not forsake them. Use your head and heart, as well as your heart and hands.

In all cases carry the symbols of your faith where you will touch them—and not just where others can read them in traffic. Practice your beliefs. And let your life be the living proof of your testament and testimony.

ᛋ Ⓢ

There are Stars in your name . . . and Sunlight. And of good forces, you will see plenty at work in your life. All you have to do is follow in the general direction, and you will find the place you're headed for. Line up your sextant to a true, fixed, and constant star, and you will not only have your mark, but you will know your coordinates.

Reading #4

1 *In the first place* you are as energetic as the fuel that you burn. Fill up on high-test, even though it's more expensive than regular unleaded, and you will get better mileage.

2 *In the second place* the real action takes place at your core. Your body is one big chemistry set. Your brain is data central. But your soul is not so easily defined. Still, you must locate, preserve, and defend it.

3 *In the third place* you come from a family cluster . . . and you need only look at your relatives to see the physical, mental, and psychological trends. Yet you must make your own magic.

In all cases the sun rises on a new day . . . every day. You can depend on it. Get into the rhythm of life. Adopt the routine, the habits, and the lifestyle that fits you.

↑ Ⓣ

There is **Triumph** in your name. So from the dust of your playing field, you are sure to emerge victorious—whatever your game. Line up your mark. Step up to the plate. Shoot for the bucket. Aim for the goal. Manage to the bottom line. Whatever you do, play to win.

1 *In the first place* you have the stamina to pump up your body and the discipline to get into shape. Take care of yourself. Stay healthy. And on the night before the big day, refrain.

2 *In the second place* you have the mental energy to psych up for the big game. Put yourself into a winning frame of mind. Don't just play the game . . . be one with it . . . be the game.

3 *In the third place* you come from a long line of contenders. These are big shoes to fill, and there is much to live up to. Thrive on the healthy competition. But if you can't beat them at their own game, challenge them to yours.

In all cases it is your winning spirit that is your claim to fame. Long after the others have quit, given up, or gone home, you're still in there slugging like a champion.

ᛒ Ⓑ

There is a breath of fresh air in your name . . . a creativity that gives you your spark. In your lifetime, you will give **B**irth to many new ideas. You will make many remarkable transitions. And of your life-altering moves, there will be almost too many to count.

❶ *In the first place* you are not afraid of hard work or of putting in the hours. Pursue your labor of love. Take your reward from the work itself. It may still pain you from time to time, but you won't really notice.

❷ *In the second place* you are able to focus. So when one of those difficult times comes, grit your teeth. Take a few deep breaths. Fixate on your focal point. And think of something beautiful.

❸ *In the third place* you want to carry on the family name. But at the very least, you will have no trouble living up to it. Carry it with pride. Keep it alive.

In all cases it is your creative energy that puts you on a growth curve. Surely your accomplishments will be recognized in their good time. And until then, *L'chaim!* my friend.

M Ⓔ

There is something f**E**male about your name. So even if you are not a woman, you are like one in a very positive way. Chances are, you can count on your feelings as well as your instincts. But I would imagine, you also know your own mind . . . and how to speak it.

❶ *In the first place* you are 100% human. So be aggressive, but not to the exclusion of civilized graces. It is better to negotiate than feud with the neighbors. Keep on speaking terms.

❷ *In the second place* you are deep, sensitive, and understanding beneath your firm surface. Don't be afraid to explore your inner mysteries. Share your mystic secrets with your trusted friends.

❸ *In the third place* you come from a long line of brave women. Honor and respect them by being brave yourself. (And don't forget to call your mother.)

In all cases the answer lies somewhere between the two extremes and his and hers. Center yourself, and you will discover your answer, as well as find some peace of mind.

ᛗ Ⓜ

There is something **Male** about your name. So even if you are not a man, you will be outwardly oriented . . . active and aggressive. You may even be ambitious. And when you get "one of those ideas" in your head, may nothing stand in your way!

1 *In the first place* you want to take the lead, get out in front, come to the head of the line, and wind up on top. But you have to fight to get ahead. So fight you must.

2 *In the second place* you are capable of acting without thinking. But remember, it takes body, mind, <u>and</u> spirit to achieve your goals. And some reflexive actions need to be controlled. Don't throw any wild punches.

3 *In the third place* you come from a long line of men who were do-do-doers. Follow their footprints like a trail in the dust. Or better yet, take to the highways they built.

In all cases you leave your mark on the world in one way or the other. "A man's gotta do what a man's gotta do." So you better get out there and do it.

ᚱ Ⓛ

There is **Love** in your name. And so, it would only seem appropriate that love should play a big part in your life. But there are many kinds of love to choose from . . . and so little time. With all you give—and all you find—there will still be plenty left to write home about.

1 *In the first place* you have to go through life trusting, rather than suspecting others. And you can't blame strangers for everything. Do your good deeds. Earn your merit badge. And forgive others their trespasses.

2 *In the second place* you have a good self-image. You are who you are. So be it. And why not? I not only like, but accept you. You might as well like yourself.

3 *In the third place* you feel a strong sense of kinship and family pride. Remain true to both your blood . . . and the in-laws. Heck, it's all one happy family around here. You might as well join in.

In all cases your cup runneth over. The more you give of love, the more there is to drink for all of us. Here's looking at you, kid. And bottoms up.

ᛉ ⓧ

Should **-ing** appear anywhere in your name, you are sure to be prolific. For **-ing** is what makes things happen. All action words are yours: Going. Doing. Being. Loving. You want to see it all, do it all, and then do it all again. What can I say but . . . I'm with you!

1 *In the first place* you are a physical being, and your body is capable of giving you pleasure. Feed it. Water it. Primp it. Pamper it. And give it a little exercise once or twice a day.

2 *In the second place* you are a sensual being. And it's hard to avoid the issue. When you see something you like, your eyes get bigger than your stomach. Try not to overindulge.

3 *In the third place* you are your parents' child. Do what comes naturally, and your line will endure and continue in more ways than one. You've got a reputation to uphold. Keep up the good work.

In all cases you accomplish what you set out to do. The choices are many. Choose among yours.

ᛟ ⑩

There is a hOme in your name . . . a dwelling place, a shelter from the cold and damp, a place to hang your hat, a place to lie down and take your rest. Everyone needs someplace to go at the end of the day. But you, especially, need to stake your claim. And your name itself gives you a handle to hold on to.

1   *In the first place* you are a natural-born nester. So put first things first. Get a ceiling over your head and put some food in the fridge. Then make your home a reflection of who you really are.

2   *In the second place* you need your own space. Starve a cold, but feed a hungry spirit. Make a nook in your place for the things you like to collect. Learn about yourself from your knickknacks.

3   *In the third place* you come from a people who found the concept of permanent shelter inviting. Hold on to what they had. Get your piece of the American pie, even if—due to inflation—it's less than 40 acres and a mule.

In all cases you fit into the place and times you find yourself. Make the most of prevailing conditions. Take advantage of how things are now.

▷◁ ⓓ

Your name spells **D**estiny, so destiny it shall be. In this life you will achieve the purpose that was meant for you. And if you don't know yet what it is, well . . . half the fun is getting there anyhow. So keep looking.

1   *In the first place* you are good at sizing up the situation and dealing with the facts. Few things are handed out, except for blessings in disguise. You'll have to unmask yours wherever you find them.

2   *In the second place* you have a sense for where you're going, and a hidden drive that will get you there. Reflect on the things you know about yourself. And act accordingly.

3   *In the third place* those who have come before you, knew what they knew. Though times have changed, the skills to deal with life are no different. Learn from the old ways.

In all cases you will seek—and find—your own truth . . . be it as it is.

0

Should you not have a first, middle or last name . . . that's **weird** indeed. But what it means is this: The fates will decide, my friend, the fates will decide. You want to take charge of your life. But certain things reside outside your control. I guess that means you'll have to work within the rules.

1   *In the first place* all the possibilities are there. And anything can happen. Prepare by being observant and attentive.

2   *In the second place* though things may not seem to have a sense of purpose, trust in the future. You'd be surprised what could yet happen.

3   *In the third place* the life you lived with your family is not necessarily the life you will make for yourself. But if the foundation is good, build on it.

In all cases you need to give things a chance to gel and settle out. Have patience, my friend. It will all coalesce in time. Have faith. It will all come together for you.

EXTRA CREDIT

To find out why you should or shouldn't do something. Name your subject. Mix up your Runes and say, ***Give me three good reasons.*** Draw three Runes at random. Or toss your Runes on the ground and then pick three without peeking.

1   **2**   **3**
1st   2nd   3rd & All
Place   Place   Cases

Look up the first Rune and read the section of the answers called "*In the first place.*" Look up your second Rune and read "*In the second place.*" Look up your third Rune and read "*In the third place.*" Also read the "*In all cases*" answer for your third Rune.

Scratch Pad

Jot down your Runes here.

EXTRA, EXTRA CREDIT!

To make a Wishing Rune. Find yourself a flat, skipping kind-of stone and paint your initials on one side. If you want to get fancy, you can combine your three Runic letters into a monogram, which was often done with Runes in the old days.

Or you can simply inscribe your stone with one of these versions of the **ING**-Rune, which according to legend will help you bring your dreams to fruition.

◈   ▷   ⬗

Make your wish and carry your lucky Rune in your purse or pocket. When your wish comes true, pitch it into a river, lake, wishing well, fountain, or woods . . . and give your troubles to the winds. (P.S. Wishing Stones make great gifts.)[1]

Go on to the next Reading whenever you are ready to continue.

---

[1] Thanks to Deon Dolphin (*Rune Magic*, NewCastle, 1987) for the idea of using a Wishing Stone.

Reading #5

WHO DO I TAKE AFTER?
(Trace my bloodline)

In this Reading, you will use the letters in your family name like Runes to learn about the family traits you inherited and the attitudes you picked up at home. Like father like son, they say . . . as mother, so daughter. Use this Reading to choose your own ways.

ᚱ ᚱ ᚱ

RUNE TOOLS

One of the first uses of Runes was for writing a person's name. All you need to perform this task is a pencil, this Reading's Scratch Pad, and the following cheat sheet. . . .

A	ᚠ	G	ᚷ	N	✝	U	ᚢ
B	ᛒ	H	ᚻ	O	ᛟ	V	ᚹ
C	ᚲ	I	ᛁ	P	ᛈ	W	ᚹ
D	ᛞ	J	ᛃ	Q	ᚲ	X	*
Ê	ᛊ	K	ᚲ	R	ᚱ	Y	ᛃ
E	ᛗ	L	ᛚ	S	ᛋ	Z	ᛉ
F	ᚠ	M	ᛗ	T	ᛏ	Th	ᚹ
'	▯	-	▯	.	▯	-ing	ᛝ

* ᛏ ᚲ ᛋ, ᚷ, or ᛉ, depending on the sound.

48

HOW TO

To learn what your family name has to say about you, just convert your name into Runes. . . .

[1]   Use the last name you were given at birth. For each letter in your family name, jot down the Rune that corresponds to it.

Scratch Pad

Jot down your Runes here.

In converting each letter of your name to Runes, there are just three tricks to remember:

- ▪ Our letter groups **Th** and **-ing** have single Runes of their own. If your name contains these groups, use the appropriate Rune, ↑ or ✕.

- ▪ There are two *E*'s. Use **M** if the sound is long, otherwise use ↓.

- ▪ Apostrophes, hyphens, periods, or blank spaces also count. If you've got one of these, add a Blank Rune to your name.

Ms. Thompson would use <u>one</u> ᚠ Rune for the first <u>two</u> letters of her name: ᚦᛜᛗᛈᛊᛜᛏ. Miss Ebert would write her <u>long</u> and <u>short</u> E's like this: ᛗᛖᛊᚱᛏ. Mr. San Giovanni would write: ᛊᚠᛏᛟᚷᛁᛜᛈᚠᛏᛏᛁ.

If you don't have your Runes yet, or if you'd just like to do a "Runeless" Reading,[1] simply look up each of your Runes now in this Reading's Answer section. Otherwise . . .

2 Sort out from your Rune stones or alphabet tiles the letters that are contained in your family names.

3 Mix up the Runes from your name. Ask: **What did my family give me?** Then draw the three Runes that call your name, and line them up in front of you.

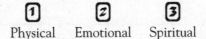

| **1** | **2** | **3** |
| Physical | Emotional | Spiritual |

The first Rune you draw indicates what your family has given you physically. The second stands for what they have given you emotionally. And the third shows what they have given you spiritually. Look up your Runes in this Reading's Answer section and read the whole answer for each, but focus on the physical, emotional, or spiritual parts, as appropriate.

THE ANSWERS

The answers appear in the traditional order of the Runes:

F U Th A R K G W H N I Y Ê P Z S T B E M L X O D

ᚠᚢ ᚦ ᚠᚱᚲᚷ ᚠᚺᚾᛏ ᛁ ᛜᛊᚲᚴᛇᛋ ᛏ ᛒᛖᛗᛗᛚ ᛥ ᛜᛞ

◻ The Blank Rune appears last.   K=C & Q; W=V; Y=J

ᚠ ◻

With **F**ortune rising out of your name, I'd say your family has given you the means to become who and what you are. In this you are for-

[1] Thank you, Rilla, for inventing the term.

tunate, my friend: Wherever your interests lie, you will find the way to pursue them. Physically, you are defined by your clothes. Emotionally, you are attached to your job. Spiritually, you are best affiliated with a group. The ends you seek are often found in real estate. Location. Location. Location. The road you are on is posted "Private Property."

∪ ⒰

With lUck jumping out of your name, I'd say you've inherited the family jewels . . . or at least the silver. In this you are charmed, my friend: You were born to the right people. Physically, you received your share of the good traits. Emotionally, you have just a few small scars to show. Spiritually, you have plenty of magic to call upon. The ends you seek are more or less handed to you. The road you are on is federally funded and state-maintained.

ᚠ ⒯ʰ

With faiTh emerging from your name, I'd say your family taught you right from wrong, all right. And—oh, boy—did you get the message! In this you are faithful, my friend: to the letter, the number, <u>and</u> the word . . . at least of your own scriptures. Physically, you like to display the signs of your belief. Emotionally, you are able to reach out and touch. Spiritually, you have your patron saints and spirit guides to contact. Whatever you achieve will be what's meant to be . . . for you. There are many paths from which to choose. Take your pick.

ᚠ ⒜

With fAte falling out of your name, I'd say your family has given you a strong sense of place. This is your fate: Whichever path you choose in the beginning brings you to the same spot in the end. Physically, you are a reflection of your self-image. Emotionally, you have plenty of props to keep your underbody stabilized. Spiritually, you are always looking for a way to improve your lot. Your course is defined by the lay of the land, by circumstance, and by precondition. The end that you seek is largely a matter of perception.

ᚱ Ⓡ

With **R**eality climbing up out of your name, I'd say your family has given you a sense of purpose. For this is your reality: You want to see everything and do it all . . . by yesterday. Physically, you are active, energetic, and outgoing. Emotionally, you are hopelessly driven. Spiritually, you are relentlessly drawn. The goal you seek is always waiting around the next bend, and you are always making up for lost time. Your life is a never-ending adventure. How could you ever be bored on this road?

ᚲ Ⓒ Ⓚ Ⓠ

With **C**ourse, **Q**uest, and **K**arma leaping from your name—all three at once—I'd say the writing on the wall was clear the day you were born. In this you are predestined: to go along for the ride. Physically, you have such big, beautiful eyes to take it all in with. Emotionally, you replay your entire life experience in sixty-second flashbacks. And spiritually, you have all the Words of Wisdom from the past. The path you are on is eternal—maybe you've even walked it before. Follow it by working with what you've ended up with this time.

ᚷ Ⓖ

With **G**ifts trailing from your name, I'd say the family has given you your fair share of everything. You are gifted, my friend, in this: You have a way of knowing how to work with the things that find their way to you. Physically, you have your fingers, toes, and other appendages to count upon. Emotionally, you are equipped with an arsenal of psychological tools. Spiritually, you are endowed with psychic skills. The ends you seek require tapping into the eternal stream. The path you are on leads to the center of things.

ᚠ Ⓥ Ⓦ

With **W**onder welling up from your name, I'd say your family gave you plenty to be glad about. You are wonderful at this: always looking on the upside, seeing the bright side, being on the light side. (Heck, you're a regular Pollyanna!) Physically, you find laughter the best medicine. Emotionally, you are able to see the humor in everything . . . even yourself. And spiritually, you know the feeling of joy welling up inside of you, until the tears run down your face. The end you seek is not entirely serious—but then again, what is? The road you are on is marked funny. (It's good to see you enjoying yourself here.)

ᚺ Ⓗ

With **H**ail falling out of your name, I'd say your family gave you your fair share of grief. Well, into every life a little rain . . . Hopefully it passed as quickly as it came. You are fortunate in this: You like your world a little stormy. Physically, you are into touch, taste, feel, and other contact sports. Emotionally, you've got a little stubborn streak or a tad of temper to watch. Spiritually, you like your Gods to talk tough once in a while. The ends that you seek depend on prevailing conditions. The road you are on is slippery when wet.

ᚾ Ⓝ

With **N**eed emerging from your name, I'd say your family has given you the tenacity to endure. In this you are never needy: You have plenty of intestinal fortitude. Physically, you are inclined to be a lean, mean, fighting machine. Emotionally, you are inventive with survival skills. And spiritually, you are better off than those who are monetarily rich. The end that you seek comes from a combination of personal sacrifice and sheer grit. The road you are on is full of potholes.

ᛁ Ⓘ

With **I**ce cropping up out of your name, I'd say your family had quite a say in shaping you . . . maybe even helping you shape up. In this you are like ice: You have become set. Physically, you have a polished surface. Emotionally, you are firm, yet inclined to be fickle. Spiritually, you tend to lock into a rigid system of beliefs . . . at least for a while. The end you seek is defined by the limits that have been set for you . . . or, more likely, that you have imposed on yourself. On the path you travel, the bridges freeze first.

◇◊ⓎⓊ

With the Year-Rune coming up out of your name, I'd say your family gave you a good work ethic. At least you understand that in order to harvest, you have to plant. In this you are perennial: You know how to rejuvenate yourself. Physically, you are quite possibly a late bloomer. Emotionally, you are as cyclical as the tides and the phases of the moon. Spiritually, you are inclined to watch out for the signs. The end that you seek comes in its own good time and proper season. The road you are on heads directly into the sun.

⌁ Ⓒ

With hElp falling from your name, I'd say your family always stood by you. And when you needed them, they were always there. In this you are aided: You have learned how to grasp the hand that is offered. Physically, you may feel fragile or dependent. Emotionally, you may know doubt. But spiritually, you can always count upon your God to bail you out. The ends that you seek are not within your single, solitary reach. But, then again, what are families for? The road you are on is lined with reflectors.

Ⓚ Ⓟ

With hoPe falling from your name, I'd say you inherited the family dream. In this you are confident: Whatever fate awaits you, you will win it fair and square. Physically, you look as good as you see yourself in the mirror. Emotionally, you are inclined to give yourself dares. And spiritually—well—you like to keep your bases covered. The road you are on may be scattered with litter and stones, but it leads to your dreams. The ends that you seek can be found with the help of Runes.

Ψ Ⓩ

With reSIStance rising in your name, I'd say your family put the fear of God in you. Why else would you be crossing yourself? In this you are blessed: Whatever evil lurks along the path, you will be bolstered by your faith. Physically, you are resilient and resistant to disease. Emotionally, you are responsive to treatment. And spiritually, you are easily convinced by the Medicine Man. The ends that you seek are good (for the most part). The path you are on is straight . . . and narrow.

⤓ Ⓢ

With **S**un & **S**tars falling from your name, I'd say your family gave it all to you . . . and more. In this you are sun-like: You never fail to rise to the moment. And if you go away, you always come back. Physically, you are fairly consistent in your game. Emotionally, you are even-tempered and for the most part predictable. Spiritually, you glow. You would look great in a halo. The end that you seek is reached by a familiar route. You know the course laid out in front of you like the back of your hand. (But still watch out for the S-curves!)

↑ Ⓣ

With **T**riumph rising from your name, I'd say your family drilled you fairly well . . . schooled you . . . and taught you the rules. In this you are triumphant: You are able to overcome your own fears. Physically, you are an athlete, champion, or warrior. Emotionally, you are a fighter—perhaps even a hero. And spiritually, you are inclined to play the role of martyr. The ends that you seek are both glorious and victorious. The road you are on is strewn with ticker tape and confetti.

ᛒ Ⓑ

With **B**irth rising from your name, I'd say your family gave you the opportunity to become yourself. This, my friend, is your birthright: You will always be true to your name. Physically, you are half your mom and half your pop. Emotionally, you are fully self-contained— but whose hang-ups did you get? Spiritually, you feel an occasional urge to break loose. The ends that you seek are self-improvements. The course you are on is labor-intensive—if not also long and hard—but well worth it.

ᛖ Ⓔ

With a fEmale rising in your name, I'd say your family taught you to respect women. In this you are feminine: You feel the answers in your heart. And you are not afraid to be sensitive. Physically, you may be soft to the touch. Emotionally, you may be unpredictable and spontaneous. But spiritually, you are deep. The ends that you seek are intuitively obvious (at least to you). The course you are on goes uphill and down.

ᛗ Ⓜ

With a Male rising in your name, I'd say your family taught you how to stand on your own two feet. In this you are like a man: You want to do things your own way. Physically, you are hard on the surface. Emotionally, you are inscrutable. And spiritually, you are quiet, but indefatigable. The ends that you seek require planning in advance. The course you are on is under construction. (Speeding fines are doubled.)

ᛚ Ⓛ

With Love bursting from your name, I'd say your family gave you the most valuable thing it could give, their love. In this way you are appreciated: They take you as you are, and—better still—they let you be. Physically, you know how to stand nice and straight. Emotionally, you have a stable base and a firm grip. And spiritually, you have managed to fit into a round hole. The ends that you seek require an ongoing commitment, but one you gladly make. The course you take from here on out is yours. It is a long and winding road.

ᛝ Ⓧ

With beING rising out of your name, I'd say you've inherited the desire to carry on the family line. In this you are blessed: You will never be for long without a bunk mate. Physically, you are attracted. Emotionally, you are enamored. And spiritually, you are connected. The ends that you desire take a little courting. But the course you are on was charted long ago. The way is as the crow flies . . . and as the bee stings.

⚒ Ⓞ

With hOme standing out from your name, I'd say your family has given you a sense of belonging. In this you are welcome: You will always have a place to go. Physically, you like to work around your digs. Emotionally, you get attached to places. And spiritually, you like to commune in the house of God. The ends that you seek—be they ever so humble—are not on the other side of the fence. The road you are on leads to your own door.

⋈ Ⓞ

With **D**estiny falling from your name, I'd say your family gave you all it needed to. The rest is up to you. You are destined in this: You have the power of choice. Physically, you go through many stages, periods, and phases. Emotionally, you weather all the changes, and even take them in stride. And spiritually, you stand in awe of the infinite Plan. The ends that you seek must be in keeping with the means. The road you are on doubles back on itself.

◻

With **weird** popping out of your name, I'd say your family didn't give you much of anything. But what's really weird is: You don't seem to expect much more. Physically, you are inclined to be rather like a chameleon. You change your appearance to suit the setting. Emotionally, you sometimes draw a blank. And spiritually, you are still looking for someone . . . something . . . or is it yourself? The course you are on is spiraling—both up and down. Be a little careful how you tread these open stairs. Draw another Rune.

EXTRA CREDIT

To trace your bloodline. Repeat this Reading using your mother's maiden name, by asking the question: **What did my mother's family give me?** Draw three Runes and consult this Reading's Answer section. Then combine your mother's Runes with the Runes of your father's name and ask, **What did I get from my parents?** You can keep going back generations if you like; just add to your pool of Runes the maiden names of your grandmothers on both sides. To trace your children's bloodline, throw in the Runes of your spouse's last name for good measure.

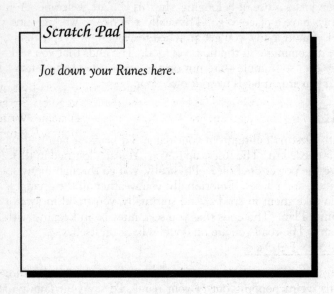

Scratch Pad

Jot down your Runes here.

EXTRA, EXTRA CREDIT!

To make Rune Staves the easy way. Get yourself 25 Popsicle sticks from your favorite hobby store. (Or what the , buy yourself a carton of freezer pops and eat your way to a set!) Once you've got your sticks, use a felt-tip marker to write one Rune on each stick, and PRESTO! you've got a fully functional set of authentic Runes staves.

To use your staves, just hold them between your hands while you think of your question. Then let go and watch them fall. Pick three from the heap and look them up in the Master Answer section of the Quick Reference Guide. Your staves will also work with any Reading in this book.

Go on to the next Reading whenever you are ready to continue.

Reading #6

WHAT ARE MY CHARMS?
(Mirror, mirror)

In this Reading, you will learn about the charming traits that make you a special character. The key is in the name you go by. So, guys, check out your nickname. Lovers, consult your pet name. Writers, look up your *nom de plume*. Hackers, try out your handle. Convicts, check your alias. Whatever name you put to it, this Reading will reveal another side of you.

<<<

RUNE TOOLS

In this Reading you will use the same tools you used in Readings #4 and #5. Here is your cheat sheet:

Letter	Rune	Letter	Rune	Letter	Rune	Letter	Rune
A	ᚠ	G	ᚷ	N	ᛏ	U	ᚢ
B	ᛒ	H	ᚺ	O	ᛟ	V	ᚡ
C	ᚲ	I	ᛁ	P	ᛈ	W	ᚹ
D	ᛗ	J	ᛃ	Q	ᚲ	X	*
Ê	ᛇ	K	ᚲ	R	ᚱ	Y	ᛃ
E	ᛖ	L	ᛚ	S	ᛋ	Z	ᛉ
F	ᚠ	M	ᛗ	T	ᛏ	Th	ᚦ
'	ᛜ	-	ᛜ	.	ᛜ	-ing	ᛜ

* ᛃ ᚲ ᛋ, ᛉ, or ᛏ, depending on the sound.

59

HOW TO

To learn what the name you go by reveals about you . . .

1 Just jot down your first name, nickname—and other aliases!—on the Scratch Pad. You can also jot down the names of those you know and love . . . anybody you care to ask about . . . anybody you want to know more about.

Scratch Pad

Jot down your names here.

---

2 Translate your name into Runes, letter for letter. Remember **Th** and **-ing** have Runes of their own. Also remember there are two E's (ᛗ as in eeny, meeny, and miney, and ᛇ as in Moe and Ed). And remember to give yourself a Blank Rune for spaces, periods, apostrophes, hyphens, and any decorative doodads you've added to your signature.

For a Runeless Reading, simply look up each of your Runes now in this Reading's Answer section. But—if you have Runes . . .

3 Separate out the Runes that are contained in your name. Mix them up while you think of the question, **What are my three**

best qualities? What makes me special? Or How am I unique?
Select the three Runes that feel familiar, and look each up in this
Reading's Answer section.

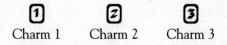

Charm 1   Charm 2   Charm 3

Each of the three will measure one of your dimensions. Try the
other names you go by, too.

THE ANSWERS

The answers appear in the traditional order of the Runes:

F U Th A R K G W H N I Y Ê P Z S T B E M L X O D

ᚠ ᚢ ᚦ ᚠ ᚱ ᚲ ᚷ ᛈ ᚺ ᚾ ᛁ ᛜᛄ ᛃ ᚲ ᛦ ᛊ ᛏ ᛒ ᛖ ᛗ ᛚ ᛉ ᛈ ᛞ

☐ **The Blank Rune appears last.** K=C & Q; W=V; Y=J

ᚠ Ⓕ

Whatever you own, my friend, it will be plenty. For you have
Fortune in your name, and its blessings are many. The F-Rune gives
you a personal magnetism. And don't be surprised if the possessions
(even persons) you seek are drawn to you as if by magic. You are
good at counting up your blessings, taking inventory of your things,
and measuring your successes by numerical means. You keep score
. . . and are usually ahead of the game. *Others see you as leading the
good life. A few are downright envious. And some are even covetous.
Choose carefully your friends, and marry wisely.*

ᚢ Ⓤ

With lUck in your name, you are inclined to seek out same. You
wear your lucky jeans . . . toss coins in a fountain . . . throw salt over
your left shoulder . . . and hold out hope that Lady Luck will stick
with you. Through thick and thin, you have eternal hope and endless dreams. And when things go in your favor, you have your lucky

stars to thank. You are a colorful character, a rugged individual, and you have no fear of going up against the odds. *Others see you as a lucky influence. They like to keep you around. But they shouldn't bet on holding you down.*

ᚠ Th

With faiTh in your name, you will be the deeply spiritual kind . . . perhaps even a zealot, fanatic, or saint. The Th-Rune draws together the trust in your heart, the hope of your spirit, and the desire of your flesh. This is powerful magic. You meditate, pray, commune, or worship as a way of manifesting your will. And if all else fails, you wait, with holy confidence, to see what your God wants. In silence and solitude you feel your way, full of faith, hope, belief, and trust in the eternal and almighty forces outside and within yourself. *Others see you as someone worthy of respect. Some even admire you. And so you must measure up to all their expectations.*

ᚠ A

The fAte-Rune in your name pretty much sums it up. You believe that what is meant to be, will be. And so be it. But you are not one to give up altogether and surrender to the whim of the fates. It's all in how you respond that counts—and you can think pretty fast on your feet. The A-Rune gives you the force to fend off a foe, to hold out for a rescue, and, in general, to survive whatever ◁ R P B hits the fan. You rise above flood, famine, and fury. You weather the winter of your discontent. But more important, you also know how to ride out a winning streak. *Others see you as one who overcomes . . . rises above . . . and makes the most of. Some even single you out as a good example for others to watch.*

ᚱ R

With Reality in your name, you will be the sort who asks the question What's it all about? . . . and then rushes off to find out. The R-Rune makes you hungry for knowledge and eager for the experience. You want to be up and doing . . . out and going . . . heave and hoeing . . . to and froing . . . live and learning. So don't be surprised if out of nowhere you suddenly get the urge to hit the road. The R-

Rune is like a Saint Christopher: It will protect you on your trip. And more important, it will guide you on your vision quest. Your calling comes to you as if on the wings of the wind. Follow the voice in your head, and it will lead you to your sure and certain truth. *Others have mixed emotions. Some encourage you. Others think you the fool out chasing windmills. Let them think what they will. And let them follow their own voices.*

< Ⓒ Ⓚ Ⓠ

The Karma-Rune in your name is a promise as much as a curse. What comes around goes around and all comes back to haunt you in the end—or so they say. But may you have pleasant dreams, my friend. For the good you give is said to come back thrice upon your own head. Keep your sights fixed on the light. (And be ever mindful of the Rule of Three.) The K-Rune gives you a sense of purpose, guidance on your lifelong Course, and sure progress in your spiritual Quest. You feel called to whatever line of work you do . . . to the people you associate with . . . the books you read . . . the CDs you play . . . and the truths you gather from these and other sources. *Others see you as someone who marches to a different beat. Some might say you are eccentric . . . erratic . . . even bizarre. But some will surely know you for what you truly are, O Enlightened One.*

✖ Ⓖ

With the G-Rune in your name, you find yourself blessed with many Gifts . . . special skills, hidden abilities, or rare and unique traits. Some of these are simply in your blood. But none of them is automatically perfected. To receive the benefits of your endowments, you may have to give something back . . . your time perhaps, your energy, your human strength. The G-Rune provides you with that warm sense of accomplishment that is, in itself, reward enough for the deed well done. But others will also say thanks. And you will never go forgotten in the minds of those you have influenced with your mere presence. *Others see you as a rare bird, an unusual beast, or an exotic creature. Some might even say you are one in a million. But I know you are one of a kind.*

ᚠ Ⓥ ᚹ

With **W**onder in your name, the world will never let you down, because the smallest things surprise and delight you. And the world is full of them. The **W**-Rune gives you a healthy sense of humor. No joke is off limits. No subject is taboo. No occasion is too sacred. In fact, the closest you ever get to drama is tragicomedy. You will never want for highlights, high points, or high moments. You find your pleasures in the most natural of things and the most common of occasions. Your life is full of enduring memories and humorous anecdotes. Besides, you relate them so well. *Others think you are the life of the party. But some would say you're "too good to be true." Still, you continue to surprise and impress them with your antics . . . as long as they continue to amuse you.*

ᚺ Ⓗ

The **H**-Rune gives you grit, my friend. For **H**ail and **H**ardship are nothing but challenges to you . . . and "no problem" . . . "no trouble" . . . "no bother" . . . and "no skin off my nose." Call the trials and tribulations of the world by whatever euphemism puts the best spin on it. This way, you'll have the attitude it takes to pass the test, endure the trial, rise above the moment, seize the finest hour, and get back up from even the lowest blow. It is your own determination that pays you back in the end. Do not be deterred by a little storm. *Though others may not always wish you well—and some may even gloat at your hard luck—you can take care of yourself. Show them what you're made of. Prove yourself to yourself.*

ᚾ Ⓝ

From **N**eed and for **N**ecessity, you grapple with the rest of them, my friend. But the **N**-Rune in your name gives you a strength and conviction that others can only envy. You hold out, make do, and get by on less than others can when times are lean and luck turns her back on you. You take nothing for granted. And as a result you generally obtain enough to satisfy your basic needs. It does not take the world to make you happy. You know how to make a little go a long way. *Others sympathize and empathize with you. They even come to your* *rescue when you are down and out. They worry about you. They care about you. And with friends like these, who needs luxury?*

I ⓘ

The I-Rune gives you Ice to overcome . . . the cold shoulder of others, the frozen heart, the rigid body, and "the way we do things around here." But Ice also melts if heated up enough. And you have the fire within you to dissolve that which is written in concrete. The fight for what you believe is right is the source of your energy, but you are the first to acknowledge the way is hard and long. Still, you are dedicated. When things start getting too deep, get out your shovel, chains, rock salt, and cat litter. *Others see you as someone who is rock-solid. But some might say you can be thick as a brick, too. Those who want to get to the real you will have to chip.*

◇ ⓨ ⓙ

The Year-Rune in your name gives you a good feeling for cause and effect. . . and an even better sense of timing. The Y-Rune helps you act and react. You are, no doubt, the type who likes to plan things out in advance. You outline the steps and the due dates. You calculate the odds for success. Nothing ventured, as they say. But in your case, you have every chance of gain. Despite the uncontrollable acts of governments and gods, this Rune gives you the foresight to plan your own life and seek your own destiny. You hold the future in your own two hands. Plant seeds now to harvest then. *Others see you as someone who believes that hard work assures success. Some are even betting on you. But others think you work too much.*

♪ ⓔ

With hElp in your name you are the sort who provides help and comfort to others . . . and gets the same in return. As you go about your deeds, the Ê-Rune protects you from forces both seen and unforeseen. It supports as you guard the welfare of others. You manage to escape unscathed from situations that are both foreboding and dangerous—and you simply seem to "ward off" disaster, as if by some magic. The truth be told, you are able to avert these threats through a combination of conviction and enthusiasm. You are a positive thinker, and this alone twists the outcome. *Others see you as someone to turn to when the chips are down. They like to hold you in reserve. And you like to come to the rescue.*

ᚹ P

The hoPe-Rune in your name gives you a good sense of the possibilities that exist . . . the options that are open . . . and the long shots that could yet come through. The **P**-Rune makes you a gambler, or at least a risk taker. At any rate, it tends to minimize your risk aversion, especially if the odds are right and the prize is good enough. When it comes to pursuing your dream, there is always a chance it's worth the risk. **P** is also the sign of fortunetellers, which helps to explain your interest in projecting the future. *Others see you as willing to put your money where your mouth is. But some would call you "a fool soon to be parted . . ." Who are you going to believe?*

ᚦ Z

The **Z**-Rune in your name gives you the resolve you need to reSISt and perSISt. "**Z**" guards your energy level and protects you . . . from weaknesses of both the physical and mental sort . . . from negative influences, which, left unchecked, would block your progress . . . and from the jealousy and ill wishes of your rivals and competitors. It is also a charm against your own lesser thoughts and bad habits. Under its shadow of protection, you are free to come and go in safety. This is your passport. *Though others might want to give you grief or cause you pain, you pass unharmed . . . even through the Slough of Despond.*

ᚴ S

The **S**un & **S**tars–Rune in your name gives you your good disposition . . . as well as your foul moods. You literally have the sun in the morning and the moon at night. And your mood swings can modulate accordingly. But the **S**-Rune also gives you a good sense of tempo and rhythm . . . keeps your biological clock in sync . . . and helps to maintain your equilibrium. You are punctual with your commitments, appointments, and designated rounds. But sometimes you have your head up in the clouds—and sometimes, too, you return to earth again. *Others see you as a ray of light in an otherwise dark Universe . . . a rising star . . . a streaking meteor. Some are even inclined to tell tall tales about you. To some you are a living legend.*

↑ Ⓣ

The T-Rune gives you Triumph, my friend . . . Triumph over the greatest odds . . . Triumph over temporary setbacks . . . Triumph over others . . . Triumph over things . . . and—last but not least—Triumph over self. For this is the Rune that protected soldiers in battle and made legends out of living men. In one way or another, you are a winner in the end, and a good sport in the process. If you would find your purpose, look for a morally justifiable cause. *Others see you as a victor and a leader. Some are looking up to you even now. Be their role model . . . you are already their hero.*

▷ Ⓑ

With **B**irth and re**B**irth in your name, you are constantly trying to better yourself, improve your condition, or advance your relative position. As the Rune that aided women in childbirth, the **B**-Rune helps you make life-altering transitions, critical passages, difficult departures, and equally emotional fresh starts. When things work against you, you are inclined to clench your fists, set your jaw, hold your breath, and bear down. Your efforts are punctuated with distinctly human sounds. *Others see you as a brave, stalwart, and dependable sort . . . even if you do complain a little bit. Some even want to bond immediately with you. (Incidentally, I like your new look.)*

M Ⓔ

The **E**-Rune gives you the power to assist others in their quest for livelihood as well as meaning in life. The **E**-Rune gives you the ability to cut to the chase and get to the point. As a result, you are regarded as a source of good advice. Others come to you seeking help, support, and certain consolation, which you are more than willing to give. There is a gentleness and compassion in your motivation and a certainty in your voice. A word from you and everything seems suddenly clear. (Why didn't I think of that?) It is your caring nature that wins the day. So even if you are not a woman, there is something wonderfully fEmale about you. (Let it all out, pal.) *Others see you as multifaceted . . . ever changing and evolving . . . a moving target to keep up with . . . and a tough act to follow.*

ᛗ Ⓜ

The Male-Rune in your name brings out the "man" in you. Even if you are a woman, there is a doggedness about you . . . and a strong spirit of independence. The **M**-Rune is like a shot of testosterone. It gives you your ambition, drive, and aggression. (And—oh yes—it also makes you want to mark your territory and occasionally go into mating frenzy.) Your primary motivation is one of conquest and control. As a result you focus your energy on altering the things around you and in gathering to you the things you need, want, and desire. In this way, you earn your place and position in the ranks of your peers. You rise above your past. You extend beyond your roots. *Others see you as a force to be reckoned with . . . a challenge as well as a threat. Some, too, are surely envious of the position you have attained. Beware the young buck. Be prepared to go stag.*

ᛚ Ⓛ

With Love in your name, you will know love's true meaning in your life, whether it comes from family, spouse, lover, child, or friend. (Heck, you may even know the love of a pet.) There are many ways and means to the same end. The **L**-Rune makes you care about others, give to others, and share yourself with others. This Rune will also make you better able to accept love from those who care about you. As such, your odds are upped for leading an all-around happy life and maybe even finding the perfect mate. The key is to open up. Reach . . . reach out . . . and touch. *Others see you as someone they can trust—even with their deepest, darkest secrets. Be sure to keep their confidences. Return their love.*

ᛝ Ⓧ

With the beING-Rune in your name, you are also lucky at love . . . at least love of a physical nature. The **ING**-Rune makes you sensuous and sensitive . . . desirous and desirable . . . attracted and attractive . . . free and available. You can't help it. You are the sort of person who is constantly aware of the sexual energy flowing through your loins. But did you know that with a little practice, you can learn how to use this energy for other creative purposes? (I didn't think so.) Abstinence and celibacy are both forms of sex, too. (But I'm with you.) Ecstasy is pretty cool. *Others pick up on you immediately. Some even pick you up. I guess you could say you're bleeping sexy.*

✠ Ⓞ

The O-Rune in your name makes you feel at hOme with your surroundings . . . the people you deal with on a daily basis . . . the situations you find yourself in. You are inclined to lead what you would call a "comfortable" existence, even if your furnishings and fixtures came cheap. What matters to you most is the company you keep and the bed you share. Though many others falsely advertise this claim, your home and family are actually "high priority" for you. All things considered, you have every reason to want to go home at the end of the day. (Can I get you a beer?) *Others like to see your headlights pulling up in the drive. Some even wave from the window. (And is that your mutt I see slavering all over you? Or do you prefer the sound of a purr?)*

⋈ Ⓓ

With the **Destiny**-Rune in your name, your own destiny is assured, for—all things considered—you will simply make it happen. The **D**-Rune is about beginnings and endings . . . starts and finishes. With this Rune operating in your name, you will make the most of the moments, hours, days, weeks, months, and years that are allotted to your purpose. And when the sun goes down, you will surely have no complaints, regrets, or desires left unfulfilled. March forward with confidence, my friend. The best is yet to be. *Others are rooting for you. Some think you are destined to do great things. And regardless of what they say to your face, they all believe in you. (And so do I.)*

Ⓞ

With the **weird**-Rune in your name, things may seem a little weird from time to time. But not to worry. It's just the Cosmic law operating in your life! It's just the great open book of your future crying out to you. It's just the way things are, were, and always shall be. This, my friend, is your fate staring you in the face. For the Blank Rune combines all the other Runes into one and puts them at your command—but when all the choices are open, the hardest thing to do is choose. Nonetheless, your path is certain. And no matter which way you turn, you cannot fail to achieve your purpose. All roads, all actions, all outcomes, and all alternatives wind up at the same end. All you have to do is lead your own life in your own way, and the rest will come naturally to you. *Others see you as being charmed, but we all know it's 99.9% perspiration.*

EXTRA CREDIT

To find out how others see you. Think of the first person you want to ask about while you mix up your Rune stones, staves, or alphabet tiles. Ask, **Mirror, mirror, tell me please, what does (so-and-so) see in me?** Reach into your bag or bowl and select three Runes. Look them up in this Reading's Answer section. Focus on the *italic* portion of the text.

1	**2**	**3**
1st	2nd	Final
Impression	Glance	Verdict

In the order you selected them, the Runes will reveal the person's first impression of you; how you appeared at second glance; and now how you look in the final verdict.

Go on to complete this Reading for the next person in your life . . . and so on and so forth.

Scratch Pad

Jot down your Runes here.

EXTRA, EXTRA CREDIT!

To make a set of money Runes. Get yourself 25 quarters ($6.25 at today's rates) and a jar of red paint. Draw a different Rune on the tail side of each coin, and you're ready to cast your fate. Your new Runes will work with any question in the book, but if your major concern is with money matters, they would seem to be ideal.

Go on to the next Reading whenever you are ready to continue.

Reading #7

WHAT'S MY SECRET TO SUCCESS?
(Whisper sweet nothings)

In this Reading, you'll learn the hidden meaning of your middle name, using the original, magical-sounding Rune names as your guides. Interestingly enough, you can also use this Reading to learn about your romantic fantasies and fetishes. It's good for a couple of laughs.

✖ ✖ ✖

RUNE TOOLS

Each Rune has an ancient name as well as a modern one. In this Reading you'll get to know the "secret" and magical-sounding names used by the ancestors:

ᚠ	Fehu	ᚺ	Hagalaz	ᛏ	Tiwaz
ᚢ	Uruz	ᚾ	Naudhiz	ᛒ	Berkano
ᚦ	Thurisaz	ᛁ	Isa	ᛗ	Ehwaz
ᚨ	Ansuz	ᛃ	Jera	ᛗ	Mannaz
ᚱ	Raidho	ᛇ	Eihwaz	ᛚ	Laguz
ᚲ	Kenaz	ᛈ	Perthro	ᛜ	Ingwaz
ᚷ	Gebo	ᛉ	Elhaz	ᛟ	Othala
ᚹ	Wunjo	ᛊ	Sowilo	ᛞ	Dagaz

72

HOW TO

To see what your middle name reveals about you . . .

1 Translate each of the letters in your middle name into Runes, using the chart in Reading #6's Tools section.

By now it should be old hat to you, but don't forget it's ▶ for **Th**, ✸ for **-ing**, ◀ for short and silent *E*, and ▶ for long *E*. Hyphens, other punctuation, and spaces in your name earn you the Blank Rune (□).

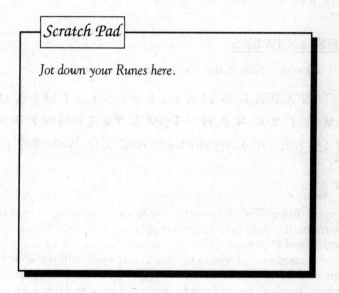

> *Scratch Pad*
>
> *Jot down your Runes here.*

For a Runeless Reading, simply look up each of your Runes now in this Reading's Answer section. To use your Runes . . .

2 Sort out the Runes in your middle name from the rest, and mix these letters together while you think of your question: **What's my secret?** to work? love? money?

3 Pick the three Runes that feel at home in your hand. Lay them faceup in a line. Then look them up in this Reading's Answer section.

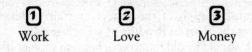

| **1** | **2** | **3** |
| Work | Love | Money |

In the order you drew them, the Runes stand for your secret to work, your secret to love, and your secret to money. Read the whole answer for each of the three, but focus on the sections that relate to work, love, and money, respectively.

THE ANSWERS

The answers appear in the traditional order of the Runes:

F U Th A R K G W H N I Y Ê P Z S T B E M L X O D

ᚠ ᚢ ᚦ ᚨ ᚱ᚜ ᚷ ᚹ ᚺᚾ ᛁ᛬ ᛃ ᛈ ᛇ ᛏᛋ ᛏ ᛒ ᛗᛘ ᛚ ᛉ ᛟᛞ

◻ The Blank Rune appears last.   K=C & Q; W=V; Y=J

ᚠ ⒡

Fortune/Fehu. With Fehu—the cow Rune—operating in your middle name, it is your herd instinct that brings you sweet success, some wealth, and even fame. Though you may need to follow in the footsteps of another—or wait your turn in line—you will rise above the rank and file in all due time. At work, you are slow but persistent. In love, you are easy and quick. With money, you account for every cent. You are artful at crafts. *You have this thing for cowhide . . . the smell of tanned leather . . . and anything wearing a belt.*

ᚢ ⒰

lUck/Uruz. With Uruz—the bull ox—operating in your middle name, it is your wild and independent nature that makes you notorious. You need to have a long leash—or at least enough rope to roam your range. At work, you are difficult to handle. In love, you like to sneak up from behind. With money, you often gamble. Your art is interactive. *You have this thing for the scent of perfume . . . flavored body oils . . . talcum . . . and musk.*

ᚠ ᚦ

faiTh/**Thurisaz**. With Thurisaz—the thorn—working in your middle name, it is your defense mechanisms that come to save the day. Nature has armed you well with the tools of survival. At work, you are quick to bare your claws. In love, you like to bite. With money, you hold on tight. And in a pinch, you summon the gods. Your art is rated PG (mild violence). *You have this thing for pierced ears . . . partially hidden tattoos . . . beauty marks . . . and, if all else fails, you're a sucker for roses.*

ᚠ ᚨ

fAte/**Ansuz**. With Ansuz—the mouth—working in your middle name, it is your way with words that gives you the upper hand. You talk fast, act quick, and fly by the seat of your pants. At work, you return calls and go to meetings. In love, you are all talk. And with money, you put it where your mouth is. Your art is rated R (adult language). *You have this thing for 1-900 numbers . . . pillow talk . . . romance stories . . . dime novels. . . and magazines with center foldouts.*

ᚱ ᚱ

Reality/**Raidho**. With Raidho—the journey—operating in your middle name, it is the experiences you've had along the way that give you your edge. You are a walking travelogue, and every story you tell has its moral. In work, you go far and wide. In love, you search high and low. And with cash—well—don't leave home without your Green Card. Your art is kinetic. *You have this thing for hotel rooms . . . do-not-disturb signs . . . room service . . . and closed-circuit movies.*

< Ⓒ Ⓚ Ⓠ

Course, Quest, Karma/Kenaz. With Kenaz—the torch—operating in your middle name, it is your 20/20 vision and your keen foresight that keeps you honed on your mark. You go through life sweeping the scene with your high beams. You even have an occasional vision. At work, you are bright. In love, you are hot to the touch. With money, you are sharp. Your art is brilliant. *You have this thing for candlelight and fireplaces . . . romantic dinners for two . . . and playing peekaboo.*

✕ Ⓖ

Gifts/Gebo. With Gebo—the gift—operating in your middle name, it is your special talents that bring you distinction. If ever in doubt, go with your intuition, hunches, and gut. At work, you are a pro at your craft. In love, you know how to make the most of flowers. And with money, you are a regular wizard. Your art is a collaborative effort. *You have this thing about getting dressed up . . . going out wining and dining . . . dancing till dawn . . . and coming home with your shoes in your hands.*

▷ Ⓥ Ⓦ

Wonder/Wunjo. With Wunjo—the joyous—operating in your middle name, it is your sense of humor that keeps you sane. When things go wrong, you have to laugh. At work, you slough it off. In love, you giggle between the sheets. And with money, it's a gas, gas, gas. Your art is a performance piece. *You have this thing about feathers . . . butterfly kisses . . . and anything else that tickles you pink.*

ⴼ Ⓗ

Hail/Hagalaz. With Hagalaz—the hailstone—striking out from your middle name, it is sheer determination that gets you through the nights. With each new Act of God that strikes, you remain firm and resolute. At work, you are a force to be reckoned with. In love, you are a tempest. And with cash, you blow it in a fury. Your art is done with special effects. *You have this thing for background noises . . .*

76

the waves on the beach . . . the rain falling on the roof . . . a train in the distance . . . the rumble of thunder.

✦ Ⓝ

Need/Naudhiz. With Naudhiz—the necessity—operating in your middle name, it is your resourcefulness that keeps gas in the tank, the utilities turned on, and the mortgage company at bay. At work, you do what you must. In love, you could handle no more than you've already got. And with money, you learn to sacrifice. Your art is surreal. *You like to imagine you are someplace else . . . with someone else . . . or that you are somebody else yourself.*

❙ Ⓘ

Ice/Isa. With Isa—the river of ice—operating in your middle name, it is your firm but slippery nature that is your hallmark. There is something going on beneath your steely surface. At work, you are hard to pin down. In love, you are cold to the touch. With money, you make solid investments. Your art is in black and white. *You have this thing for cold showers . . . piping hot baths . . . and playing foot-sie under the covers.*

◇ Ⓨ Ⓙ

Year/Jera. With Jera—the cycle of the year—operating in your middle name, it is your ability to plan ahead that gets you done on deadline. Plant, water, and tend your garden. Prayer does the rest, and the flowers come. With work, it will be seasonal. At love, you will be fruitful. And with cash, it will be paid back when the crops come in. Your art is the landscape itself. *You have this thing for getting dirty . . . making love in the great outdoors . . . or waiting until the moon is full.*

♪ Ⓔ

hElp/Eihwaz. With Eihwaz—the yew tree—operating in your middle name, it is your evergreen nature that distinguishes you. You have a secret reserve of inner strength that gives you vitality. At work, you are stalwart. In love, you are constant and true. With money, you are able to stretch it out and make it do. Your art is rated PG-13. *You have this thing about personal hygiene . . . blood tests . . . condoms . . . and (who knows) maybe even surgical gloves.*

hoPe/Perthro. With Perthro—the dice cup—operating in your middle name, it is your willingness to bet on the future that changes everything. You put all you can on the line. At work, you bet your life. In love, you crawl out on a limb. And with money, you let it ride. Your art is all in the wrist. *You have this thing for chance encounters . . . strangers in a strange land . . . ships that pass in the night . . . and a good old-fashioned game of Russian roulette.*

reSIStance/Elhaz. With Elhaz—the antlers of an elk—operating in your middle name, it is your ability to butt heads with the opposition that wins you the game. You believe in yourself. You trust in your God. At work, you charge in. In love, you barge in. And with money—well—you sure do know the value of a buck. Your art is an African print. *You have this thing for deep breathing . . . primal screaming . . . animal noises . . . and anything else that sounds unmistakably like the call of the wild.*

Sun & Stars/Sowilo. With Sowilo—the sun wheel—operating in your middle name, you are always ready to roll. You rise, shine, and get on the road. At work, you spend your days. In love, you pass your nights. And with money, you must earn, earn, earn to pay, pay, pay. Your art is as childlike as a Picasso. *You have this thing for tan lines . . . swimsuits . . . wet T-shirts . . . skinny-dips . . . and a friendly game of volleyball on the beach.*

Triumph/Tiwaz. With Tiwaz—the warrior—operating in your middle name, it is by skill, strategy, and savoir faire that you come out the winner. At work, you are a regular trooper. In love, you ride the high command. And with money—well—you'd best see the pay-master. Your art is rated R (for language, nudity, and lack of plot). *You have this thing for athletic gear . . . personnel in uniform . . . short hair . . . and someone who knows how to handle a weapon.*

ᛒ Ⓑ

Birth/Berkano. With Berkano—the birches—operating in your middle name, it is your way of bending in the breeze that gives you flexibility. Try to remain limber and nimble as life sweeps over and around you. Your work is a labor of love. Your love is something you work at. And your money comes and goes . . . goes and comes. Your art is a work in progress. *You have this thing for new positions . . . new roles . . . new games . . . and you are always in the market for new toys.*

M Ⓔ

fEmale/Ehwaz. With Ehwaz—the mare—operating in your middle name, it is your unbridled spirit and your tame heart that combine to win you the race. You are a mixture of strength and grace. At work, you team up. In love, you don't mind the idea of being hitched. And with money, you have a hay day. Your art is made with bold strokes of the brush. *You have this thing for jeans, spurs, and cowboy boots . . . hats . . . chaps . . . and (I don't know) maybe even a buggy whip.*

ᛗ Ⓜ

Male/Mannaz. With Mannaz—the man—operating in your middle name, it is your blood, sweat, and tears that sway the world to your way of thinking. At work, you are a wolf in sheep's clothing. In love, you're always on the prowl. And with money—well—it's something you can really sink your teeth in. Your art is done with special tools. *You have this thing for camcorders . . . remote control . . . freeze-frame video . . . clever little gadgets . . . and anything that operates off batteries.*

ᚱ Ⓛ

Love/Laguz. With Laguz—the water—operating in your middle name, it is your ability to go with the flow that allows you to always fit in. Life can be as easy as floating on your back. At work, things get done before you know it. In love, it all comes naturally. And with money, there is a steady flow of green. Your art is a love song. *You have this thing for shimmering swimming pools . . . spume-swept beaches . . . white-water rivers . . . Old Faithful . . . Niagara Falls . . . and anything else that gushes.*

ᚼ Ⓧ

beING/Ingwaz. With Ingwaz—the fertility god—operating in your middle name, it is your personal magnetism—and the glint in your eye—that is your claim to fame. At work, you are a distraction. In love, you really know how to attract 'em. And when it comes to money, others are always picking up your tab. Your art is rated triple X. *You have this thing for explicit talk . . . full frontal nudity . . . adult situations . . . and tight (albeit fuzzy) close-ups on the action.*

ᚼ Ⓞ

hOme/Othala. With Othala—the land of the ancestors—operating in your middle name, it is your sense of family that gives you both your purpose and your sense of pride. You are one of the clan. At work, you sign on for the duration. In love, you try to make it last forever. And with money, you help out all the rest. Your art is a family photograph on the desk. *You have this thing for flannel pajamas . . . snacking in bed . . . and coming home for lunch some days.*

ᛞ Ⓓ

Destiny/Dagaz. With Dagaz—the day—operating in your middle name, it is your sense of time and place that brings you safely to your goal. At work you are there when they need you. In love, you fit it in, morning, noon, and night. And with money, the time till pay-day has a way of passing fast. Your art is a sunset. *You have this thing* *for putting out the cat . . . turning out the lights . . . and crawling naked between the sheets.*

O

weird. With **weird** operating in your middle name, it is "those crazy coincidences" that seem to shape your life. Things have a way of just happening to you. At work, you just fall into your job. In love, you just keep bumping into one another. And with money, a little extra always comes just in time. Your art is spontaneous. *You have this thing for photo finishes . . . flash performances . . . quickies . . . and anything that can be done in ten minutes or less.*

EXTRA CREDIT

To find out what you have a "thing" for. For an interesting diversion—and a few laughs at your next party—here's a provocative little game you can play with your friends. Just gather everyone together in a circle. Give your Runes a good mixing up. Then say, **Whisper our sweet nothings**. Pass your Runes around and have everyone choose one. Look each person's Rune up in this Reading's Answer section and read the *italic* portion of the text. To liven things up, add this rule: If your Rune doesn't quite describe your real fetish, fantasy, or hang-up—well then—just tell the circle what does.

EXTRA, EXTRA CREDIT!

How to make traditional Rune lots. To do this craft project, you need a bunch of wooden nickels, old buttons, or circles cut from cardboard. For the woodworker, get yourself a dowel stick, an old chair leg, or a tree branch that's about two or three feet long and about an inch or so in diameter. Put on your goggles and saw the wood into segments that are about $3/4$ inch thick. You'll need 25 chips (nickels, buttons, or circles) in all. Carve, paint, or woodburn a Rune on each slice.

To use your lots, wait for the paint to dry. Then ask any question on your mind. Draw the three Runes that call your name, and put them in a line. Look up your Runes in the Master Answer section of the Quick Reference Guide. Read the whole answer for each, but focus on the sections of the text that relate to your question (Work, Love, Money, or—for most other questions—Strategy). Your lots will also work with any Reading in the book.

Go on to the next Reading whenever you are ready to continue.

Reading #8

HOW SHOULD I PROCEED?
(Show me my choices)

_____

In this Reading, you will use your Runes or alphabet tiles to seek direction on any matter that concerns you . . . relationships, jobs, finances, politics . . . or just about anything that requires resolution in your world right now.

ᚠ ᚠ ᚠ

RUNE TOOLS

The traditional way to read Runes is three at a time. In interpreting your answers, the secret lies in the order that the Runes are selected (❶ , ❷ , ❸) and in the way that each position in the three-Rune layout has been "preprogrammed"—defined and set—by the user. The three positions can be set to just about any three things you can think of. In the last few Readings, we've programmed them variously as . . .

❶	❷	❸
1st Thing	2nd Thing	3rd Thing
Past	Present	Future
Physical	Emotional	Spiritual
Work	Love	Money

In this Reading we'll be programming them in yet another way, which has grown increasingly popular of late and is a good problem-solving approach: Situation, Action, and Result.

HOW TO

To see how you should proceed in whatever course of endeavor you choose . . .

[1] Mix up your Runes or alphabet tiles while you think of your question: **How should I proceed?** in my job hunt? my love affairs? my marriage? my work? Or simply **What must I do?**

[2] Now, with your question in mind, reach into your Runes and select the first Rune that "feels right." Or cast your Runes on the floor and select one at random. Place it faceup in front of you. Draw two more Runes in the same way, and line them up, left to right.

Scratch Pad

Jot down your Runes here.

---

[3] Look up your Runes in this Reading's Answer section.

Situation **Action** **Result**

The first Rune you selected stands for the situation you are currently in. The second stands for the action you should take to make things go your way. And finally, the third Rune tells you what will be achieved as a result of taking this action.

Since these answers have been written to handle all types of questions, you may need to read between the lines a bit and draw your own conclusions. For more detail on any Rune, look it up in the Master Answer section.

THE ANSWERS

The answers appear in the traditional order of the Runes:

F U Th A R K G W H N I Y Ê P Z S T B E M L X O D

ᚠ ᚢ ᚦ ᚨ ᚱ ᚲ ᚷ ᚹ ᚺ ᚾ ᛁ ᛃ ᛈ ᛉ ᛊ ᛏ ᛒ ᛖ ᛗ ᛚ ᛜ ᛟ

☐ The Blank Rune appears last. K=C & Q; W=V; Y=J

ᚠ Ⓕ

Fortune/Fehu/Cow

Situation. You live in a green meadow of cash on the hoof . . . and only an occasional cow pie. You live in a world where you can count upon the things that money buys. *Action.* Head 'em up. Move 'em out. Let the buyer beware. Glance back over your shoulder. Watch where you step. "There is so much good in the worst of us, and so much bad in the best of us."[1] *Result.* The market fluctuates. Fortunes come and go, like fads. Friends turn fairweathered. The falcon circles slowly in the clear blue air . . . looking for carrion.

[1] Edward Wallis Hoch (1849–1928)

U Ⓤ

lUck/Uruz/Bull

Situation. You live in a world where things tend to go your way—at least in sudden fits and bursts. You roam your range, mark its boundary limits, and have your pick of the herd. *Action.* Keep going where you're going. Keep doing what you're doing. At the first sign of danger, assume a defensive stance. And whatever you do, don't ⊠ Ⓤ ◁ ◁ with a winning streak. "Have but luck and you will have the rest."[2] *Result.* Your luck changes—and may it be from good to best! You ride out the winning streak. You wait out the temporary downturn. You make your comeback. The bull lowers its head and paws at the dust.

ᚦ Ⓣⓗ

faiTh/Thurisaz/Thorn

Situation. You are living in an imperfect world, where things sometimes go wrong for no apparent rhyme or reason and where bad things happen to good people. It seems you have been thrown into the bramble patch. *Action.* Muster all the faith you have left. Summon your God to the cause. By sheer determination and inner resolve, untangle the knots that tie you down. Pull out the barbs. *Result.* The thorn has drawn its blood for the day. You live, learn, and go forth to trust again. Say your thanks. "All things work together for good to them that love God."[3]

ᚨ Ⓐ

fAte/Ansuz/Mouth

Situation. You live in a world where words count, especially if they are brief and to the point. Everybody is talking so fast, you can

[2] Victor Hugo, *Les Misérables* (1862)
[3] Romans 8:28, King James Bible

hardly think. Yet nobody ever says anything. And hardly anyone listens. *Action*. Be all ears, but keep all pacts. Guard the tricks of the trade. And speak no trash. *Result*. The word comes. You can believe what you hear from someone close to the source. You heed your own familiar voice. The mouth curves its edges up in a Mona Lisa smile. "In the beginning was the Word," my friend. "And the Word <u>was</u> God."[4]

ᚱ ®

Reality/Raidho/Journey

Situation. You live in a world that grows smaller every day. The wide road stretches out in front of you like an airstrip. Something at a distance beckons with a sweeping light among the clouds. You look beyond the horizon. *Action*. Go where you must. Do all you can. See all there is to see. Learn all there is to ken. "Life is not measured by the time we live."[5] *Result*. Here you go again! You follow the call of your wild. And eventually it will bring you back from the wilderness . . . just as surely as it took you there in the first place.

ᚲ ⓒ ⓚ ⓠ

Course, Quest, Karma/Kenaz/Torch

Situation. There is something that lights up your world—a candle in the window . . . a spark in the heart. Suddenly the mists that obscured your path lift. You have seen a vision. *Action*. Light a lamp. Aim your flashlight. Turn on your headlights . . . and be 20% more visible. *Result*. Your light is a beacon for others. What they see in you is a reflection of the promise you offer them. "The torch has been passed to a new generation."[6]

---

[4] John 1:1, King James Bible
[5] Rev. George Crabbe (1783)
[6] John F. Kennedy, Inaugural Address, 1961

✕ ☉

Gifts/Gebo/Gift

Situation. You are living in a world of artists, inventors, dreamers . . . idealists and their ideas. You yourself have many thoughts to give and many sentiments to share. *Action*. Develop your skills. Perfect your techniques. Practice your craft. Improvise. Innovate. But most of all, Trust your precognition. "Having gifts that differ . . . let us use them: If prophecy, in proportion to our faith."[7] *Result*. Gifts are exchanged. Favors are traded. A social engagement is attended. You take them a present. (What a nice gesture.)

ᚠ ⋁ ⋀

Wonder/Wunjo/Joy

Situation. You are feeling on top of your world. Everything is going your way. And it makes a ✕ ᚠ ✕ ☉ good story. You feel appreciated and liked. *Action*. Keep your sense of humor with you at all times. Take a joke. Get your kicks however you can. And whistle while you work. *Result*. Everyone is tickled pink, especially you. You have the last (and best) laugh of all. A little bundle arrives at your doorstep. "Joy delights in joy."[8]

ᚺ ⊞

Hail/Hagalaz/Hail

Situation. Your world is a disaster zone right now. The environment is disturbing. And Mother Nature is brewing up a few surprises of her own. There may even be hellfire and brimstone before this storm is come and gone. *Action*. Seek shelter at the first sign of threatening conditions. Heed all warnings. And follow all illuminated placards. Pack your rubbers. *Result*. It all blows over in the end. Things calm down . . . and everything returns to normal. You

---

[7] Romans 12:6, Revised Standard Bible
[8] William Shakespeare, *Sonnets*: VIII (1609)

pick up the pieces and carry on. Even hail the size of golf balls melts soon after it falls. "Faith can stifle all science."[9]

✦ Ⓝ

Need/Naudhiz/Need

Situation. Your world's been looking pretty sparse and spare of late. And you're feeling pretty down and out and fairly hard up. Well, to make a breakthrough always causes a little angst. *Action.* Stand by, my friend. Lie low. Hide out. Await your cue that the coast is clear. Then, with care, stick your neck out. *Result.* There is more to be gained than lost in this. You end up making a little sacrifice . . . but so what? "If of thy mortal goods thou art bereft . . . buy hyacinths to feed thy soul."[10]

▌ Ⓘ

Ice/Isa/Ice

Situation. The world can be a bitter place sometimes. The north wind sweeps down, and from the south comes freezing rain. Things grind to a halt, and nobody's getting anywhere fast on the interstate. *Action.* Call it a day. Shut down. Wall up. Settle in for the duration. Let it snow, let it snow, let it snow. *Result.* These things have a way of dissolving. It will all be forgotten in a couple of nights. And looking back, it will have all been only a petty aggravation. "Deliver me from the oppression of man."[11]

◇ Ⓨ Ⓙ

Year/Jera/Year

Situation. This is a world where nothing lasts forever and nothing stays the same for very long. Both good and bad have—at best—

---

[9] H. F. Amiel, Journal, Feb. 7, 1872
[10] Gulistan of Moslih Eddin Saadi, 13th century Persian poet
[11] Psalm 119:134, King James Bible (*FYI: This Psalm has a stanza for every letter of the Hebrew alphabet*)

their seasons. Enjoy it while it lasts . . . or else count the days until it will be past. *Action*. Time things out. Await the proper place and the right moment. Make a date. Meet when the moon is ripe. *Result*. You finish what you start. You market what you make. You are what you eat. You become what you did. "Should auld acquaintance be forgot."[12]

♪ Ⓔ

hElp/Eihwaz/Yew

Situation. You live in a frightening, intimidating world, subject to disease, disaster, and occasional death. And, it seems, there is a constant struggle going on between "good" and "evil." May the guys in the white hats win. *Action*. Ready your rebuttal. Put up your dukes. Radio for backup. Call in the guard. *Result*. A miracle occurs. Help comes. You are delivered from danger. The yew springs back after a winter storm. "The Lord is my shepherd, I shall not want."[13]

𐌊 Ⓟ

hoPe/Perthro/Dice Cup

Situation. Your world is a risky place, where only Lloyds will cover all the bets. All around you people are gambling. All around you people are wishing to win at the game. *Action*. Read the tip sheet. Calculate the spread. Go with your hunches. And place your bets in time—don't get shut out, my friend. *Result*. Sometimes ya wins, sometimes ya loses. But this time, you quit while you're ahead. The dice skitter across the green felt. "Luck is one half of success."[14]

[12] Robert Burns, "Auld Lang Syne"
[13] Psalm 23, King James Bible
[14] Hindu proverb

ᛉ Ⓩ

reSIStance/Elhaz/Elk

Situation. You live in a world of disease, plague, drought, pestilence, and medical politics. You find yourself among folk who would sell your soul to drink from the Fountain of Youth. *Action*. Take your high-priced medication as directed. But lobby for human decency in your healthier moments. Uphold the Bill of Rights. Keep the Golden Rule. *Result*. The surgeon general regards you as a clear and present danger. The lone elk in musk bellows to the moon. "The Devil can cite scripture for his purpose."[15]

ᛋ Ⓢ

Sun & Stars/Sowilo/Sun

Situation. You live in a world decorated with sun, moon, and stars . . . and punctuated by those scattered, random, few-and-far-between moments that take your breath away. This is one of those times made for snapshots. *Action*. Hold on to the night. Embrace the dawn of a new day. Make a wish on the evening star. Count your blessings. *Result*. Wow! What an experience. (I think I felt the earth move!) It must have been in the stars. "And let them be for signs and for seasons and for days and for years."[16]

ᛏ Ⓣ

Triumph/Tiwaz/The Warrior

Situation. You live in a world of wars, strike forces, and peace-keeping troops. You live in a world with rumors of unrest. And soon you may be called upon to fight. *Action*. Rise to the challenge. Gird your loins. Paint Runes on the shaft of your spear. ᛏ ᛏ ᛏ . *Result*. You emerge from this battle triumphant, but changed. The hero brushes

---

[15] Shakespeare, *Merchant of Venice*, Act 1, Scene 3
[16] Genesis 1:14, the Creation Story, King James Bible

the confetti from his brow, waves his hand, and steps back down into the crowd. "And the people shall answer and say Amen."[17]

ᛒ Ⓑ

Birth/Berkano/Birches

Situation. You live in a world where the rules were made to be bent—especially your rules, especially by you. Nothing ever happens the same way twice. No two births are ever alike. And you can't learn another soul's lesson. *Action.* Boil water. Rend cloth. Call in a Wise Woman. Carve Runes into bark. ᛒ ᛒ ᛒ. *Result.* Congratulations. (Sneak out back with me, and we'll have a smoke.) The spring winds have scattered a gazillion seeds on the walk. And the spring rains have come along to plant the ones that fell on good soil. "We believe whatever we want to believe."[18]

ᛗ Ⓔ

fEmale/Ehwaz/The Mare

Situation. You live in a woman's world, where the feelings of others count as equal to the job that needs done. Things get handled by committee. Everyone has a vote. It's a win/win situation, if I ever saw one. *Action.* Attend the meeting. Consult with your peers. Assign tasks. Get organized. *Result.* Everything comes together at last. All the pieces fall into place. Everyone did her part. And everyone shares in the credit. "Her ways are ways of pleasantness and all her paths are peace."[19]

ᛗ Ⓜ

[17] Deuteronomy 17:15, King James Bible
[18] Demosthenes (348 B.C.)
[19] Proverbs 3:17, King James Bible

92

Male/Mannaz/Man

Situation. You live in a man's world. Everyone has a job to do. Things get done as a team. But the captain calls the shots. It's a win-or-lose situation, all right. *Action.* Listen to the boss. Follow orders. Fall in line. Pull your own weight. *Result.* Everything shapes up according to plan. Everyone moves in the same general direction. Everyone gets his share of the glory . . . and the pain. "What is man that thou art mindful of him."[20]

ᚱ ᛚ

Love/Laguz/Water

Situation. You live in a world of calm surfaces, but strong undertows and swift currents. You live in a world where the tides change with the moon and where emotions run high and low—in about the same pattern. But you love it, don't you? *Action.* Consult your charts. Sound out the surrounding depths. Pay attention to your dreams. Drink lots of fluids. Get plenty of sleep. *Result.* You'll be feeling yourself again in a few days. The message becomes clear at Full Moon. "Many waters cannot quench love, nor floods drown it."[21]

ᛜ ᛝ

beING/Ingwaz/Sex

Situation. You live in a world of mutually consenting adults, gender issues, and sexual politics. You live in a time when people kiss and tell the morning audience. What do they have on you? *Action.* Orient yourself however you like. And respect the rights and privacy of others to do the same. Do your part to preserve the species: Use condoms. *Result.* You could find yourself having sex on a more regular basis. "Let us go out early to the vineyards. . . . There will I give you my love."[22]

[20] Psalm 8:4, King James Bible
[21] Song of Songs (which is Solomon's) 8:7, Revised Standard Bible
[22] Song of Songs 7:12, Revised Standard Bible

✖ Ⓞ

hOme/Othala/Homeland

Situation. You live in a world of your own making. You live with your own people and the things you have collected. You lead your own life. *Action.* Set your own hours. Eat when you're hungry. Shave if you want. Bathe if you like. And throw another log on the fire. *Result.* You click your ruby-red slippers once, twice, thrice. "We hold these truths to be self-evident."[23] There's no place like home. Enjoy your day off.

✖ Ⓓ

Destiny/Dagaz/Day

Situation. You live in a world that goes from one extreme to the other . . . and it seems as if the rules have changed overnight. What once was okay is not always all right. It just depends on how the law is read . . . and by what kind of person. "Give me liberty or give me death."[24] *Action.* Quietly, seek safety in numbers. Wait until you see the pendulum swing back again. Then seize your day. "Proclaim liberty throughout the land."[25] *Result.* Everything comes back around in time. And everything old is new again. "Weeping may endure for a night, but joy cometh in the morning."[26]

Ⓞ

weird

Situation. You live in a world where the leaders wear makeup. You live in a place where science is religion . . . and church is state. You live in a time when people are encouraged to turn each other in. The future cannot be seen for the chaos of the present. *Action.* Wipe the slate clean. Get back to basics. Assert your indepen-

---

[23] Declaration of Independence, July 4, 1776
[24] Patrick Henry's speech before the Virginia Convention, 1775
[25] Inscription on the Liberty Bell, Philadelphia, Pennsylvania
[26] Psalms 30:5, King James Bible

dence. Exercise the rights given you by the Powers of Nature. *Result.* It all lies in your own two hands. Uphold the Founding Fathers' dream. "The enumeration of certain rights shall not be construed to deny or disparage others retained by the people."[27]

EXTRA CREDIT

To *explore choices*. Mix up your Runes and ask, **Show me my options** with regard to _____? Select three Runes. And look them up in this Reading's Answer section. For each Rune, read the portion of the text that is listed after *"Action."* These are the three possibilities you should consider. Take your question on to Reading #9's Extra Credit section to explore which option would be best to pursue.

EXTRA, EXTRA CREDIT!

Adopt a tree. Some of the Runes we have been working with are traditionally associated with trees. Now's your chance to save one—by dedicating it to someone you love. Just separate out the following six Runes from your set: ᚠ ᛃ ᚲ ᚦ ᛒ ᚠ. Think of your love. Say, **Carve my love's initials.** Select one Rune. Here's what it means:

ᚠ **Oak.** Tie a yellow ribbon, my friend, and await. Adopt this Rune for a love so strong, it can hardly stand to be separated.

ᛃ **Yew.** Push up new shoots, my friend. Renew your vows. Adopt this Rune for a love that can endure the test of time.

ᚲ **Apple.** An apple a day, my pretty. So take your pick. Adopt this Rune for the love that's chosen over all the rest.

ᚦ **Hawthorn.** Drape garlands, my friend. And hang a wreath on the door. Adopt this Rune for a love that is chaste, loyal, and pure.

[27] The Constitution of the United States of America, Bill of Rights, Article 9, 1787

ⓔ **Birch.** Stand tall, my friend. Stand out white against the forest. Adopt this Rune for a love rooted with commitment.

ⓕ **Ash.** Sink your roots deep, my friend. And stay for the duration. Adopt this Rune for the love that was always meant to be.

Go on to the next Reading whenever you are ready to continue.

Reading #9

WHAT IF . . . ?
(Answer me twice)

In this Reading you will use your Runes to consider the various options open to you. What if you take that new job? What if you move to a new place? What if you make that "sure" investment? What if . . .

НННН

RUNE TOOLS

Up until now, we have been reading our Runes from left to right just as we read and write English now. . . .

1　　　**2**　　　**3**

But in the early days of Runes there were no such rules. Sometimes Runes were written right to left, just like letters in Hebrew. It's also possible to read and write them that way now, if you prefer. . . .

3　　　**2**　　　**1**

To show you how it feels, this Reading performs a special trick that gives you an answer both frontwards <u>and</u> backwards!

HOW TO

To evaluate your choices . . .

1　　Mix up your Runes while you think of your question. **What if I decide to** _____? quit my job? move out West? sell my house? **What if I decide <u>not</u> to** _____? marry? move? switch jobs? invest? The Reading works for most anything you drop in the blank.

② Then, with your question in mind, reach into your Runes and select three that feel promising. Or cast a big handful of Runes on the floor and select three. Line up the Runes you have selected faceup either from left to right or right to left.

Scratch Pad

Jot down your Runes here.

---

③ The fun comes when you start to look up your answers. For each Rune, the Answer section contains some text followed by a chart listing the other 24 Runes. Here's how to read your answers. . . .

Rune 1—Read the main text, look up Rune 2 in the chart.

Rune 2—Read the main text, look up Rune 3 in the chart.

Rune 3—Read the main text, look up Rune 2 in the chart.

Rune 2—Read the main text, look up Rune 1 in the chart.

The answer you receive from reading your Runes in this way is inclined to be a "circular argument." You will either get the same answer when you read your Runes frontwards and backwards, or you might get two alternative views of the same situation—but both will be correct.

For more details on any Rune, turn to the Master Answer section.

THE ANSWERS

The answers appear in the traditional order of the Runes:

F U Th A R K G W H N I Y Ê P Z S T B E M L X O D

ᚠᚢ ᚦᚨ ᚱ< ᚷᚹ ᚺᚾ ᛁᛇᛸᛚᛝᛦ ᛊᛏ ᛒᛖᛗ ᛞᛚᛜᛟ

O   The Blank Rune appears last.   K=C & Q; W=V; Y=J

ᚠ Ⓕ

Fortune—When the money side of things works out for you, the books can be balanced, your accounts squared away, your worldly goods and chattel numbered, and your estate planned. When paired with other Runes, it tells you what kind of success you will have. . . .

ᚠ F ———		ᚺ H	A storm is avoided.
ᚢ U You luck out.		ᚾ N	A period of difficulty ends.
ᚦ Th You get religion.			
ᚨ A A debt is paid back.		ᛁ I	Things get locked up.
ᚱ R A journey is fortuitous.		ᛸ Y	The time goes fast.
< K A flame is kindled.		ᛚ Ê	Help arrives.
ᚷ G A gift is given.		ᛝ P	A risk pays off.
ᚹ W Joy leaps in your breast.		ᛦ Z	Danger is averted.

S   The weather holds up.

T   Victory is won.

B   A birth is recorded.

E   You win over a woman.

M   You win over a man.

L   Love wins over everything.

X   The earth moves.

O   A home is built.

D   Your day comes.

O   You have it your way.

lUck

lUck—When your luck holds up, a few little things go a long way. A Guardian Angel looks out for you. A Good Samaritan comes by. You happen to be in the right place at the right time. When paired with other Runes, it indicates the kind of chance you will get . . .

F   The chance to prosper

U   ——————

Th The chance to aspire

A   The chance to inspire

R   The chance to go far and wide

K   The chance to shine

G   The chance to open up

W   The chance to enjoy life

H   The chance to persist

N   The chance to survive

I   The chance to change

Y   The chance to complete

Ê   The chance to help out

P   The chance to play your hand

Z   The chance to escape

S   The chance to get some color

T   The chance to compete

ᛒ B The chance to start all over

ᛗ E The chance to meet a woman

ᛗ M The chance to meet a man

ᛚ L The chance to show you care

� X The chance to couple

ᛜ O The chance to stay at home

ᛞ D The chance to be fulfilled

ᛟ The chance of a lifetime

ᚦ ⓣₕ

fai**TH**—When you have faith, everything goes according to a higher plan. Everything has a purpose, place, and time. Everything has a reason and a rhyme. All the pieces fall into place. And there is no such thing as coincidence. When paired with other Runes, it shows who in your life is being blessed right now . . .

ᚠ F Blessed are the owners.

ᚢ U Blessed are the players.

ᚦ Th ———

ᚨ A Blessed are the outcasts.

ᚱ R Blessed are the wayfarers.

ᚲ K Blessed are the enlightened.

ᚷ G Blessed are the givers.

ᚹ W Blessed are those who laugh.

ᚺ H Blessed are those who weep.

ᚾ N Blessed are the poor.

ᛁ I Blessed are the pure in heart.

ᛃ Y Blessed are those who labor.

ᛇ Ê Blessed are the troubled.

ᛈ P Blessed are the risk takers.

ᛉ Z Blessed are the healthy.

ᛋ S Blessed are the stars.

ᛏ T Blessed are the heroes.

ᛒ B Blessed are the newborn.

ᛗ E Blessed is the woman.

ᛗ M Blessed is the man.

ᛚ L Blessed is love.

ᛉ X Blessed is sex.

ᛟ O Blessed is the dwelling place.

ᛞ D Blessed are the days.

ᛯ Blessed be.

ᚠ ⒜

fAte—When fate is on your side, things can go either way. It just depends. Were you good boys and girls this year? Or will Santa bring you a lump of coal for your stocking? Things have a way of evening out in this Universe of ours. When paired with other Runes, it shows which fate awaits you . . .

ᚠ F A fortuitous decision

ᚢ U A lucky break

ᚦ Th A predestined event

ᚠ A ———

ᚱ R A fateful journey

ᚲ K A light at the end of the tunnel

ᚷ G A gift from the gods

ᚹ W A couple of laughs

ᚺ H A great big adventure

ᛏ N A good, long cry

ᛁ I A test of endurance

ᛃ Y A year to work and wait

ᛇ Ê An ordeal to pass through

ᛈ P A winner to pick

ᛉ Z A test of faith

ᛋ S An act of assurance

102

ᛏ T A fight to the finish

ᛒ B A rite of passage

ᛖ E A woman to test

ᛗ M A man to test

ᛚ L A love to prove

ᛝ X Two ships that pass

ᛟ O A homecoming

ᛞ D A day to remember

▯ A blank check

ᚱ Ⓡ

Reality—When reality comes into play, it's time for a sanity check. Weigh the pros and cons, add plus to minus, list out strengths, confess to weaknesses. Is this really what you want to do? Only you can tell. Search out the truth, and then you'll know. When paired with other Runes, it indicates the type of mission you are on . . .

ᚠ F A cattle drive

ᚢ U A wild-goose chase

ᚦ Th A pilgrimage

ᚨ A An eternal quest

ᚱ R ———

ᚲ K A command performance

ᚷ G A diplomatic mission

ᚹ W A shot at happiness

ᚺ H A stint of hazardous duty

ᚾ N A supply mission

ᛁ I An ice-cutting maneuver

ᛃ Y A complete tour of active duty

ᛇ Ê A rescue mission

ᛈ P A pipe dream

ᛉ Z A counterstrike

ᛊ S A shot in the dark

ᛏ T An heroic attempt

ᛒ B A deliverance

M E A woman's issue

M M A man's thing

ᚱ L A love affair

ᚷ X A sexual conquest

ᛟ O A family matter

M D A full day's wages

☐ A journey of a thousand days

ᚲ © Ⓚ ℚ

Course, Quest, Karma—With these three operating as one in your life, you will feel things start to click. There is a call you must answer and a light you must see. Once the voice is heeded, the way walked, and the deed done, you will see what your light has revealed. When paired with other Runes, it indicates the form your vision will take . . .

ᚠ F An illusion

ᚢ U A vivid dream

ᚦ Th A prophetic utterance

ᚨ A A flashback in time

ᚱ R A shimmering mirage

ᚲ K ———

ᚷ G A sudden inspiration

ᚹ W A hallucination

ᚺ H A blinding flash

ᛏ N A sign in the embers

ᛁ I A cold shiver

ᛃ Y A déjà vu

ᛇ Ê A smoke signal

ᛈ P A message from the Runes

ᛉ Z A graphic symbol

ᛋ S A sign in the sky

ᛏ T An instant replay

ᛒ B A rude awakening

ᛗ E   A premonition   ᛆ X   A hot flash

ᛘ M   A lucky hunch   ᛉ O   An apparition

ᚱ L   A good feeling   ᛝ D   A daydream

ᛜ   Let your mind go blank.

ᚷ G

Gifts—When gifts like these drop into your lap, you have nothing to do but thank your lucky stars . . . and unwrap. All that you need comes to you in a silver stream. This is your opportunity to celebrate. When paired with other Runes, it gives you a hint about the surprise that's coming . . .

ᚠ F   A windfall   ᛁ I   A change in temperature

ᚢ U   A piece of cake   ᛇ Y   A twist at the end

ᚦ Th A knock on the door   ᛃ Ê   A welcome assist

ᚨ A   An ironic twist   ᛈ P   Instant winnings

ᚱ R   A spontaneous trip   ᛉ Z   A secret weapon

ᚲ K   A sudden realization ᛊ S   A total eclipse

ᚷ G   ———   ᛏ T   A surprise attack

ᚹ W   An unsuspected punch   ᛒ B   A special delivery
      line
                           ᛗ E   A gift horse
ᚺ H   A temporary falling out

ᚾ N   A booby prize   ᛘ M   A slap on the back

▶ L A peck on the cheek   ✖ O A housewarming gift

✖ X A mark on the neck   ▷◁ D An hour back come fall

▢ A big surprise

▶ Ⓥ ⱳ

Wonder—When a sense of wonder fills your life, you look at things as if you've never seen them before. This is a fairy-tale ending to a most enchanting story. I guess there is something new under the sun, after all. And relatively speaking, there must be a first time for everything. When paired with other Runes, it indicates the kind of thrill you can expect . . .

ᚠ F A steak dinner   ᛁ I Goose bumps

ᚢ U A trip to the bank   ᚤ Y A sense of
                                   accomplishment

ᚦ Th A charismatic
      experience   ᛇ Ê A sigh of relief

ᚠ A A past life regression ᚹ P Instant gratification

ᚱ R An out-of-body flight   ᛉ Z A rush of adrenaline

ᚲ K A creative download   ᛋ S A Rocky Mountain high

✖ G A package in the mail   ᛏ T A victory dance

ᚹ W ——   ᛒ B A breath of fresh air

ᚻ H Thrills and chills   ᛗ E A bareback ride

ᛏ N Pins and needles   ▷◁ M Zero to 60 in nothing
                                    flat

ᛚ L A scented note   ᛟ O A burnt mortgage

ᛜ X A 10 on the Richter   ᛞ D A day off with pay
       scale

ᛜ A thrill a minute

ᚺ ⊕

Hail—When hail shows up in your life, it means Mother Nature is up to her old tricks. You can expect to see high winds, rough seas, and bending trees. A period of difficulty is within radar range. But behind it, the skies are clear. When paired with other Runes, it indicates the kind of trouble you must try to prevent . . .

ᚠ F Money trouble   ᛁ I Freezing rain and flash
                                     floods

ᚢ U Tough luck   ᛇ Y Wasted time

ᚦ Th A moment of doubt   ᛖ Ê The good intention

ᚨ A A past-due note   ᛈ P A losing streak

ᚱ R Hazardous driving   ᛉ Z A battle of nerves
       conditions

ᚲ K Power outages, energy   ᛊ S Overexposure
       surges

ᚷ G A bribe or kickback   ᛏ T A battle of wills

ᚹ W A battle of wits   ᛒ B Labor disputes

ᚺ H ———   ᛗ E Woman troubles

ᚾ N Double trouble   ᛘ M Man troubles

107

ᚱ L Lovers' spats   ᛟ O Faulty construction

ᛉ X Impotence   ᛞ D The day of reckoning

      ᛜ Inclement weather

ᚾ ⓝ

Need—When need enters into things, the struggle intensifies. It's time to separate the men from the boys and the women from the girls. It's time to beat the chaff from the wheat. How resourceful can you be? Let's see. Paired with other Runes, it indicates your most important need . . .

ᚠ F To trade the cow for magic beans

ᚢ U To pull a plum from your pie

ᚦ Th To keep your platter clean

ᚨ A To sing heigh-ho, heigh-ho

ᚱ R To leave a trail of bread crumbs

ᚲ K To jump over the candlestick

ᚷ G To put a ring on your finger

ᚹ W To wear bells on your toes

ᚺ H To feel the wind in your topknot

ᚾ N ————

ᛁ I To slide upon the ice

ᛇ Y To keep the garden free of weeds

ᛈ Ê To puzzle the Rule of Three

ᛈ P To unscramble the riddle

ᛉ Z To turn 'em out knaves all three

ᛊ S To sweep the cobwebs from the sky

ᛏ T To gunpowder, reason, and plot

ᛒ B To whip them all soundly

ᛗ E To be sugar, spice, everything nice

ᛗ M To be frogs, snails, puppy dog tails

ᛋ X To go rub-a-dub-dub

ᛟ O To share a cup of ale

ᛚ L To count kits, cats, sacks, wives

ᛞ D To make hay while the sun shines

ᛟ Hark! Hark! The dogs do bark![1]

ᛁ ᛟ

Ice—When ice forms in your life, everything is sealed, reinforced, locked in, and tightened up. So jockey for position and then settle into your place. Things will remain just as they are long enough to catch your breath. When combined with other Runes, it indicates that you can expect something to be on hold for a while . . .

ᚠ F Your liquid assets

ᚢ U Your current run of luck

ᚦ Th Your humble petition

ᚨ A Your tongue in your cheek

ᚱ R Domestic travel plans

ᚲ K A back-burnered idea

ᚷ G A diamond ring

ᚹ W The last laugh

ᚺ H A planned outing

ᛜ N A few frills

ᛁ I ———

ᛇ Y A return on investment

ᛃ Ê A Christmas fund

ᛈ P Your winnings

ᛉ Z A plan of attack

ᛋ S A summer vacation

ᛏ T A score to settle

ᛒ B A big commitment

ᛗ E A new wardrobe

ᛗ M A better car

[1] With thanks to Mother Goose

Γ L A standing relationship   **⋈** O A new house

⋈ X Casual sex   **▷◁** D A deadline

◻ Just about everything

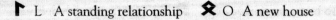

Year—When the Year Rune shows up, it will take a year or 13 moons for things to work out. Give your ideas the time they need to sprout, develop, and mature. Things have a way of working out in 52 weeks (or 365 days). Give things a full turning of the seasons to be resolved. When paired with other Runes, it indicates the type of payback you can expect . . .

Γ F Top dollar   **I** I A flood of emotions

U U Double your money   **◇** Y _____

Þ Th The answer to a silent prayer **♪** Ê A favor returned

Γ A A suspended sentence   **Κ** P A free spin

R R A return trip   **Ψ** Z A period of grace

< K A long-term goal achieved   **S** S A beautiful tan

X G A beautiful reward   **↑** T A coveted honor

Γ W A reason to smile   **B** B A fresh start

H H A timely deliverance   **M** E The woman of your dreams

↑ N A penny for your thoughts   **⋈** M The man you desire

110

| ┌ L A love that lasts | ⊗ O The home you make of it |
| ⊠ X Your kind of sex | ⋈ D A return to normalcy |

☐ You make the call.

♪ Ê

hElp—When help shows up in your life, it's always a welcome relief, but especially at the moment when it's needed most. The bad news is, there is some reason to call for it. You need to be on the alert, if not also on the defensive. Don't hesitate to ask for assistance. When paired with other Runes, it indicates your best defense is to . . .

F F Borrow from equity.	**I** I Go out on strike.
U U Carry a Rune in your pocket.	**Y** Y Turn the other cheek.
Þ Th Feast before you fast.	**♪** Ê ——
A A Watch your mouth.	**P** P Check the dice before you roll.
R R See the guru.	**Z** Z Just say no.
K K Light a candle.	**S** S Wear sunscreen number 15.
G G Make a sacrifice.	**T** T Send for reinforcements.
W W Get high on life.	**B** B Listen to your coach.
H H Rail at the Universe.	**E** E See the woman.
N N Ask for relief.	**M** M See the man.

111

ᛚ L Turn to your love.   ᛟ O Ask your family.

ᛉ X Make a new friend.   ᛞ D Go to bed.

ᛁ Cry HELP!

ᚲ (ᛟ)

hoPe—When hope comes to the fore, it boosts your confidence and gives you cause to look ahead. You reach into the Runes and take your pick, knowing that the fate in store for you is worth the knowing in advance. Why be frightened of the future? When paired with other Runes, it tells you what to hold out hope for . . .

ᚠ F The jackpot   ᛁ I A rock-solid reason

ᚢ U A streak of good luck   ᛇ Y A great season

ᚦ Th Plenty of loaves and fishes   ᛃ Ê A miracle cure

ᚨ A Better luck next time   ᚲ P ———

ᚱ R Happy trails   ᛉ Z A moral victory

ᚲ K A look on the bright side   ᛋ S A giant leap

    ᛏ T A timely rescue

ᚷ G A baker's dozen   ᛒ B A safe passage

ᚹ W A laugh a minute   ᛗ E An equal say

ᚺ H A walk on the wild side   ᛗ M A fair play

ᚾ N A need satisfied   ᛚ L A lifelong friendship

✖ X A lasting love affair   ▶◀ D A great life

✖ O A place of your own

◻ Anything and everything

Ψ ⓩ

re**SIS**tance—When resistance shows up in your life, the good news is, you will be protected. The question is, what is it you need to be protected from? And is it real or imagined?' When paired with other Runes, it tells you what you need to resist . . .

ᚠ F The root of all evil   ᛐ Ê Fear of the unknown

ᚢ U A change of heart   ᚹ P A false hope

ᚦ Th The work of the devil   Ψ Z ——————

ᚨ A A fatalistic attitude   ᛋ S Mercury in retrograde

ᚱ R A false prophecy   ᛏ T Campaign promises

ᚲ K The powers of darkness   ᛒ B A selfish wish

ᚷ G Propaganda   ᛖ E A Trojan horse

ᚹ W The temptation to laugh   ▶◀ M The Wolfman

ᚺ H A confrontation   ᚴ L An unwelcome advance

ᚾ N A poisoned dart   ✖ X Exchanging body fluids

ᛁ I Frostbite   ✖ O A money pit

ᛦ Y Forcing a thing too soon   ▶◀ D Waiting until it's too late

◻ A feeling of uncertainty

ᛋ Ⓢ

Sun & Stars—With the sun, moon, and stars lighting up your life, there's really not much more to say. This is one of those perfect opportunities that only comes along every now and again. So before the Concorde leaves the jetway, you'd better get on board. When paired with other Runes, it indicates the nature of the opportunity at hand . . .

ᚠ F A top-flight company

ᚢ U A fast track to success

ᚦ Th A ticket to paradise

ᚨ A A ground-floor opportunity

ᚱ R A long-haul proposition

ᚲ K A golden opportunity

ᚷ G A good trade-off

ᚹ W A happy compromise

ᚺ H A challenging situation

ᚾ N A real challenging situation

ᛁ I A short-term proposition

ᛇ Y A one-year contract

ᛃ Ê A trial period

ᛈ P A calculated risk

ᛉ Z A permanent assignment

ᛋ S _____

ᛏ T A power play

ᛒ B A start-up operation

ᛖ E An equal opportunity

ᛗ M An open-and-shut case

ᛚ L A joint venture

ᛜ X A passion play

ᛜ O An opportunity to work at home

ᛞ D An ongoing arrangement

ᛟ Keep your options open.

ᛏ (T)

Triumph—When triumph shows up in your Runes, you can expect to win at whatever you are attempting to do. In this contest, your best weapons are stamina and finesse. Your proper performance only improves under pressure. When paired with other Runes, it tells you how close a victory it will be . . .

ᚠ F By a landslide

ᚢ U By a hair's width

ᚦ Th In the final seconds

ᚨ A By the skin of your teeth

ᚱ R By a mile

ᚲ K A photo finish

ᚷ G A tie

ᚹ W A runaway hit

ᚺ H A close call

ᚾ N A knockout

ᛁ I A slim margin

ᛃ Y In overtime

ᛇ Ê Down to the wire

ᛈ P By a coin toss

ᛉ Z On a wing and a prayer

ᛊ S At the speed of light

ᛏ T ———

ᛒ B By a few centimeters

ᛖ E By a neck

ᛗ M By six inches

ᛚ L By a heartbeat

ᛜ X Close enough to taste

ᛟ O By a few yards

ᛞ D By the end of the day

□ No contest

ᛒ (B)

Birth—When birth turns up in your Runes, you can expect that your life will change overnight. You take on new roles, duties, and responsibilities. Your life has new meaning; and you, a new sense of purpose. When paired with other Runes, it describes the kind of birth or rebirth it will be . . .

ᚠ	F	A physical change	ᛐ	Ê	An assisted delivery
ᚢ	U	An easy transition	ᚴ	P	Head over heels
ᚦ	Th	A spiritual reawakening	ᚤ	Z	Fist in glove
ᚨ	A	A progressive step	ᛋ	S	A supernova
ᚱ	R	A different line of work	ᛏ	T	A test of bravery
ᚲ	K	A mystical experience	ᛒ	B	———
ᚷ	G	A new talent to show	ᛗ	E	A resolution
ᚹ	W	A fresh stab at happiness	ᛙ	M	An initiation
ᚺ	H	A rude awakening	ᛚ	L	A test of loyalty
ᛏ	N	A trial by fire	ᛩ	X	A sensual awakening
ᛁ	I	A psychological ordeal	ᛪ	O	A consecration
ᛤ	Y	A coming-of-age	ᛞ	D	A coming-to-terms

ᛟ   A brand new life

ᛗⒺ

fEmale—When the female is operating in your life, you will know the right thing to do as you do it. But don't be surprised if you also get some advance notice in the form of a sign to read or a symbol to interpret. When paired with other Runes, it gives you an omen to ponder . . .

ᚠ	F	A penny found	ᚦ	Th✚	
ᚢ	U	A penny lost	ᚨ	A	Chickens to count

R R A black cat in the way

K K Three on a match

G G "Do not open until Christmas"

W W Laughter at a funeral

H H A red sky in morning

N N Friday the 13th

I I Yellow snow

Y Y A blue moon

Ê Ê ⊘

P P Cards cut three times

Z Z ☮

S S A falling star

T T A white flag

B B A silver spoon

E E ——

M M ♂ ♀

L L The clock's upswing

X X Never on a Sunday

O O 🧍 🧍 🧍 🐕

D D The stroke of midnight

O Take it as a good sign.

M Ⓜ

Male—When a male influence enters your life, you'll need to stake out the playing field and establish the ground rules. But not so fast—because not just anybody is allowed to play. Before you can get on the team, you must be initiated. When paired with other Runes, it indicates what you'll have to do to get into the club . . .

F F Pay your dues.

U U Take the dare.

Th Th Get through hell week.

A A Assume your place in rank.

R R Run the gauntlet.

K K Pass the torch.

X G Give 'em all you've got.

P W Laugh at their jokes.

H H Brave the elements.

+ N Be their whipping boy.

I I Play the scapegoat.

<> Y Put in the time.

J Ê Don't let 'em see you sweat.

K P Don't let 'em call your bluff.

Y Z Don't let on you're scared.

S S Get up at the crack of dawn.

↑ T Pass the physical challenge.

B B Write your name in blood.

M E Ride bareback.

M M _____

Γ L Kiss someone's ass.

X X Talk in expletives.

◇ O Give the secret password.

M D Pull an all-nighter.

O Be your own "man."

⌐⊙

Love—When love conquers all, there will be no pretending anymore. And you can throw your black book out with the trash. Love occurs beneath the surface. There is no test—you will simply know when it is right. When paired with other Runes, it shows the love you get this time around . . .

F F You love to leave your mark.

U U You love to play pick up.

P Th You love to feign innocence.

R A You love to feel guilty.

118

ᚱ R You love to go, go, go.

ᚲ K You love to play with fire.

ᚷ G You love to untie bows.

ᚹ W You love to get your jollies.

ᚺ H You love to throw stones.

ᚾ N You love a sad ending.

ᛁ I You love feeling stranded.

ᛃ Y You love a Harvest Moon.

ᛇ Ê You love to moan about it.

ᛈ P You love to tease.

ᛉ Z You love to squeeze.

ᛋ S You love to see stars.

ᛏ T You love your land.

ᛒ B You love your kin.

ᛖ E You love a woman.

ᛗ M You love a man.

ᛚ L _____

ᛜ X You love to roll in the hay.

ᛟ O You love to play house.

ᛞ D You love a spring day.

ᛜ The love of your life finds you.

ᛜᛝ

beING—When your sexual being shows up, it's a sign that things are about to happen for you. The steam is building. The temperature is rising. Your heart is racing lickety-splickety. And your breath is coming in pants. When paired with other Runes, it indicates the type of energy burst you can expect . . .

ᚠ F An all-out stampede

ᚢ U A multiple climax

ᚦ Th A slow dissolve to black

ᚨ A A second wind

R   A train going into a tunnel

K   A rocket blasting off

G   A cork popping

W   A scream of delight

H   A white tornado

N   A fireworks display

I   The head on a beer

Y   Waves crashing on the beach

Ê   A delayed response

P   A chain reaction

Z   A quick discharge

S   A slow progression of events

T   A slam dunk

B   A race to the finish

E   A flurry of activity

M   A ten-minute workout

L   A passionate display

X   ———

O   A home run

D   A sunrise dripping with gold

  A quiet release

hOme—When home is on your mind, nothing much else matters. For this is the place where heart, body, and soul reside. Be it ever so humble. This is the place that when you go there, you want to stay forever and ever. When paired with other Runes, it tells what kind of place you will have . . .

F   A money pit

U   A place that's free and clear

Th   A humble abode

A   The place you deserve

R   A pup tent

K   A house of mirrors

✕ G A gift house

ᚹ W At least you can laugh about it.

ᚺ H A weather-beaten, old place

✝ N A fixer-upper

❙ I An igloo

❖ Y A year-round residence

◢ Ê A sanctuary

ᚴ P A pool parlor

ᚼ Z A haunted house

ᔕ S A summer place

↑ T A barracks

ᛒ B A nursery

ᛗ E A place with a woman's touch

ᛗ M A place needing a woman's touch

ᚱ L A place you adore

✖ X A love nest

✕ O ———

ᛞ D A house that is a home

◻ Anyplace you like

ᛞ◻

Destiny—When destiny rears its lovely head, you'll know it's simply meant to be. Day in, day out, the wheels are in motion. And you can hardly get off the carousel now. Look sharp. Here comes the brass ring. When paired with other Runes, it reveals what you have come to learn . . .

ᚠ F Only you can tell your fortune.

ᚢ U Only you can trust your luck.

ᚦ Th Only you can show your faith.

ᚨ A Only you can pass your test.

ᚱ R Only you can seek your truth.

ᚲ K Only you can find your light.

✖ G Only you can use your gifts.

▶ W Only you can dance your dance.

╟ H Only you can give 'em hell.

✝ N Only you can do your best.

▌ I Only you can melt their hearts.

✦ Y Only you can save the crops.

↲ Ê Only you can cry for help.

⬚ P Only you can put up the stakes.

Ψ Z Only you can stand 'em off.

◆ S Only you can reach your top.

↑ T Only you can win your fight.

B B Only you can claim your rights.

M E Only you can know for sure.

M M Only you can give the proof.

Γ L Only you can feel it too.

❈ X Only you can do it like you do.

✖ O Only you can find your niche.

▶◀ D ——

☐ Only you can save the day.

☐

weird—When things turn weird on you, anything can happen (and often does). It's either a funny coincidence or something totally off the wall. Watch for the unexpected to occur. It comes at you from left field. It falls from out of the blue. When paired with other Runes, it indicates "something strange" . . .

ᚠ F Funny money

ᚢ U An odd sequence of
events

ᚦ Th Strange occurrences

ᚨ A Flashbacks to a former
life

ᚱ R A feeling of inertia

ᚲ K Mixed signals

ᚷ G Crossed purposes

ᚹ W A riddle to solve

ᚻ H An unpredictable event

ᚾ N A nagging feeling

ᛁ I A shiver down the back

ᛄ Y A sudden change of pace

ᛇ Ê A feeling of anxiety

ᛈ P A sudden impulse

ᛉ Z A wariness

ᛋ S A strange light in the
sky

ᛏ T A feeling of doom

ᛒ B An expectancy

ᛖ E A strange woman

ᛗ M A strange man

ᛚ L A strange love

᛬ X A stranger

ᛜ O A strange place

ᛞ D A strange day

ᛟ _____

EXTRA CREDIT

Double-barreled questions. To consider two courses of action at
once, mix up your Runes while you think of the decision you are trying to make. With your issue in mind, ask, **What if I do and what
if I don't?** Or simply, **Answer me twice.** Select six Runes, and
arrange them into a horseshoe. . . .

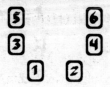

Runes 1, 3, and 5 will answer the what-if-you-do portion of the question, and Runes 2, 4, and 6 will answer the what-if-you-don't portion. Look up your Runes in this Reading's Answer section and read the main text. (For kicks, you can also look up adjacent Runes in the charts following the main text.)

The layout also works in considering two different options at once: What if I go to Company X and what if I start my own business?

EXTRA, EXTRA CREDIT!

How to make Rune stones—the easy way. Get yourself 25 relatively flat pebbles of about the same size (an inch or so in diameter is good). Beach pebbles come to mind, or you might have luck at your local creek, run, or streambed. City dwellers, visit your local craft store or New Age shop. Once you've got your stones, use paint, indelible ink, or a felt-tip marker to paint on the Runes, one Rune to a stone. Paint the Rune on one side only, leaving the opposite side blank. Once you have written all the Runes, you will be left with one blank stone. For a personal touch, sign your name and write the date on this one. (And don't forget, Rune stones are another great gift-giving idea.)

Go on to the next Reading whenever you are ready to continue.

Reading #10

What Are My Needs?

(Tell me when the moon is right)

In this Reading you will use the day you were born to identify your "birthstone" Rune, which in turn will reveal a little bit about your basic needs. Or you can also use this Reading to draw or cast your Runes in order to determine which day of the month would favor a particular type of activity or action.

RUNE TOOLS

It's likely that sometimes you will draw a Rune and turn it over to find its Runic letter upside down: ᚠ ᚢ ᚦ ᚨ ᚱ ᚲ. The same goes for your alphabet tiles, of course: ∀ ꓭ Ͻ ᗡ Ǝ Ⅎ ⅁. As you might have guessed, Runes that are "in reversal" have a different meaning from their upright counterparts.

The "calendar" that we're going to be using for this Reading makes use of all the Runes that can be reversed. Ten Runes (ᚷ, ᚺ, ᚾ, ᛁ, ᛜ, ᛇ, ᛊ, ᛃ, ᛞ, and ☐) don't look any different upside down, so they have no reversed meanings and do not appear reversed in the chart.

THE RUNES AND THEIR DAYS

	Day	Rune Sign		Day	Rune Sign
	FRI	ᚠ		4th	ᚨ
☽	1st	ᚠ		5th	ᚨ
	2nd	ᚢ		6th	ᚨ
	3rd	ᚢ		7th	ᚱ
	THU	ᚦ	◑	8th	ᚱ

	Day	Rune Sign		Day	Rune Sign
	9th	ᐸ		TUE	↑
	10th	ᐳ	◖	22nd	↓
◖	11th	✕		B-day	ᛒ
	WED	ᚠ		23rd	ᛃ
	12th	ᛈ		24th	ᛘ
	H-day	ᚺ		25th	ᛠ
	13th	✝		MON	ᛩ
	14th	ᛁ		26th	ᛪ
◖	15th	ᛆ		27th	ᚱ
	16th	ᛐ		28th	ᛒ
	17th	ᛰ	◖	29th	ᛮ
◖	18th	ᛉ		SUN	ᛮ
	19th	ᛦ		SAT	ᛮ
	20th	ᛐ	▢	30th	ᛤ
	21st	ᛋ		31st	▯

Since this assignment of Runes is based on the phases of the moon,[1] I've included moons in the chart. They will come in handy for those who do the Extra, Extra Credit portion of this Reading.

HOW TO

To learn what the day you were born says about you . . .

1   Look up the <u>day of the month</u> that you were born in the preceding chart (or consult the chart for the dates of those who matter most to you).

[1] Thanks to Michael Erlwine for his insights on lunar astrology ("Lunar Gaps: Taking Advantage of the Moon Cycle," <u>Matrix Journal</u>, Vol. 2, Issue 1, 1990).

There are three additional tricks you can try . . .

- Look up the <u>day of the week</u> (Monday, Tuesday . . .) that the birth took place. If you don't know what day it was, consult the chart for "B-day."

- If you were born on or within three days of a holiday, consult the chart for "H-day."

- If you know what the phase of the moon was on that day, look that up too.

②   Copy down the Rune that appears next to your day. If your Rune is upside down, copy it upside down.

Scratch Pad

Jot down your Runes here.

③   Look up your Runes (right side up or upside down) in this Reading's Answer section.

This Reading will also handle questions like **What do I need?** with regard to a job? a love? Or **What is my world like?** at work?

at home? Just mix up your Runes, ask your question, and draw one, two, or three Runes.

THE ANSWERS

The answers appear in the traditional order of the Runes, with reversals immediately following their upright counterparts.

F U Th A R K G W H N I Y Ê P Z S T B E M L X O D

ᚠᚢᚦᚨᚱᚲᚷᚹᚺᚾᛁᛃᛇᛈᛉᛊᛏᛒᛖᛗᛚᛜᛟᛞ

☐ The Blank Rune appears last.   K=C & Q; W=V; Y=J

ᚠ Ⓕ

Fortune.   Friday's child, 'tis said, is full of woe.[2]   No greater lie was ever told.   For Friday is a blessed day, when the work of the week ends and everyone goes home a little early.   You need to make a living, but you don't need to kill yourself for the company, do you? *Make it till Friday night.   Wait for payday.*   ☐ *When the Crescent Moon appears briefly at sunset, it's time to boogie.*

ᚡ Ⓕ

Fortune reversed.   Sad but true, you need money to do the things you want to do.   For it is money that gives you true freedom in this world of ours.   It is money that conveys the status others admire, and it is money that gives you the buying power.   *The first of the month is good for starters.*   ☐ *Wait to act until you see the Crescent Moon at dusk.*

ᚢ Ⓤ

lUck.   You need to feel as if you've got a chance to get ahead.   For without a little luck, no one ever succeeds.   You need your charms, birthstones, lucky numbers, daily horoscopes, or favorite supersti-

---

[2] The answers for the days of the week are based loosely on the traditional folk poem "Birthdays," as quoted in *Bartlett's Familiar Quotations*, 12th edition, p. 1,068.

tions to get you psyched. Whatever works for you. *The 2nd is the day to launch projects.* ◲ *Keep an eye out at sunset for the horns of a wishing moon. Then make one.*

ᚾ ⓝ

lUck reversed. You need your luck to change. But—lucky you—it always does. No one stays on top for long. No one remains on the bottom forever. You need to watch out for your big breaks, that's all. You need to seize the opportunity when it knocks. *The 3rd will be your lucky day.* ◲ *Watch for the Crescent Moon that trails behind the sun.*

ᚦ ⓣʰ

faiTh. Thursday's child works hard, they say. For life is thorny. And the roses are brief, few, and far between upon the barbed stem. The way is narrow. The going is grief. Who would have more perfect need for faith than these? *By Thursday you will have your sign.* ◲ *Take heart when the Crescent Moon stays into night.*

ᚨ ⓣʰ

faiTh reversed. You need something to keep your spirits high. For this is a world where people struggle—even in this day and age, and regardless of their rank or holy station. You need your prayers, hymns, litanies, rosaries, or scripture verses to keep you going. You need your Sunday morning dose of endorphins. *What happens on the 4th will be a blessing in disguise.* ◲ *Gather your courage as the Crescent Moon grows and gathers strength.*

ᚠ Ⓐ

fAte. You need to be encouraged. For nothing in this world of ours gets done unless there is a prize at the end. You need your periodic pats on the back and an occasional word of thanks, not to mention recompense. *By the 5th, you will receive your just reward.* ◲ *As the Crescent Moon fills, ask what you will.*

↓ Ⓥ

fAte reversed. You need to be forgiven. No one can be held totally responsible for what a lifetime brings. And no one has ever
walked this far without getting a blister. Justice may be blind, but a
judge must be all-seeing. You need to be excused. You need to be
pardoned. *The 6th is a good day to ask for permission.* ◗ *As the moon
approaches the quarter, the tides grow still.*

◤ Ⓡ

Reality. You need to follow your own drummer. For reality is nothing but relative, and each individual is unique. You need to have
some space. You need to establish some distance. You need to
express yourself. You need to develop your own interests. *The 7th
is your lucky day.* ◗ *As the Quarter Moon comes, listen for your call.*

↓ Ⓝ

Reality reversed. You need to compromise. For this is a world of
square pegs, round holes, and oddballs. You need to fit into the
scheme of things somehow, and yet not lose your very soul in the
process. *Make a date for the 8th.* ◗ *Watch, wait, and listen to your
instincts on the night when the Quarter Moon shines bright.*

◀ Ⓒ Ⓚ Ⓠ

Course, Quest, Karma. You need to take the high road. For even
in this cosmetic and hypocritical world of ours, the truth is a torch.
You need to speak out for human dignity, or else risk losing your
own. You need to follow your star. *Go on the 9th.* ◗ *Feel your heart
stir as the Quarter Moon builds.*

▶ Ⓒ Ⓝ Ⓞ

Course, Quest, Karma reversed. You need to take the low road. For
even in this land of the free and this home of the brave, you run the
risk of sticking your neck out too far. You need to support what is
politically correct for a while. You need to give in to popular belief,
or else be hammered into place. *Set aside the 10th to remember.* ◗
As the Quarter Moon waxes, honor the founder of the feast.

✕ Ⓖ Ⓖ

Gifts. You need to use your gifts. Even in this high-tech world of ours, there is a need for artists. You need to sing, dance, paint, write, sculpt, compose . . . CREATE. You need to tap into the cosmic stream. You need to use your psychic abilities. You need to trust your feelings. *Something wonderful comes to you on the 11th.* ◒ *Pay attention to your dreams as the moon waxes to Full.*

Ⓟ Ⓥ Ⓦ

Wonder. Wednesday's child, the old rhymes say, loves much, gives more, knows joy instead of sorrow, and wears the look of wonder in its eye. 'Tis true. There is much to marvel at and thrill over. You need not even look too hard for the rainbow. *By Wednesday you will be over the hump for sure.* ◒ *Feel your spirit start to soar as the moon builds . . . and builds.*

◀ Ⓐ Ⓦ

Wonder reversed. You need to keep your secrets to yourself. For even in a world where artists are welcome, certain subjects are taboo. You need to go underground and wait for these generations to pass and for time to prove whose work was genius. *I'd go with 12th night.* ◒ *When you can see the woman's profile in the moon, you will have your sign.*

Ⓗ Ⓗ

Hail. Those born to a holiday are tied to it in certain ways that only they can know for sure. It all depends on which day it is and how it falls this year. A mixed blessing, at best. A minor curse, at worst. You need to establish your own identity. *Wait until after the holidays.* ◒ *As the moon turns full, turn inward.*

✝ Ⓝ

Need. You really need it bad! For in this world of haves and have-nots, sometimes you get, and sometimes you don't. We all need to fast as well as feast. We all need to restrain in order to indulge. And you need to celebrate as well as sacrifice. *Don't back off from the 13th. But don't press your luck either.* ◙ *When the moon waxes fuller and fuller, it's time to give up a little something. Make a penance.*

| ⓘ

Ice. You need to loosen up. For even in this rigid world of ours, the rules can be bent. You need to be firm yet flexible. You need to be hard yet soft. You need to put a little glide into your skates. *The 14th looks good to me. But be sensitive.* ◙ *The emotional tides run both hot and cold, as the moon grows full.*

◇ Ⓨ Ⓐ Ⓙ ⓡ

Year. You need to do things according to your inner clock. For even in this world of calendars, schedules, and timepieces, there is a place for syncopation. Dance to your own rhythm, even if it varies from the norm . . . even if it has a few extra notes, or skips a beat from time to time. *And just you wait till the Ides!* ◙ *Make note of your feelings at the Full Moon. Get together with a kindred spirit. See the man. Watch for an eclipse.*

↑ Ⓔ Ⓔ

hElp. You need help . . . but, then again, who doesn't? For in this crazy, mixed-up world, who's to say who's normal and who's not? You need to muster your faith and courage, and—above all else—believe in yourself. You need to take the risk of being considered eccentric. *The 16th will be your salvation.* ◙ *Count your blessings when the moon rises full for the second night running.*

Ⓚ Ⓟ

hoPe. You need to keep up your spirits. For in this world where magical things <u>do</u> occur, someone's dream comes true every seventeen seconds. You have as good a chance as any, especially if you believe miracles can happen . . . to you. *The 17th will prove you can.* ◙ *As the Full Moon wanes, you will feel it in your bones.*

⋈ ⓙ

hoPe reversed. You need to know when to quit. For in this world where some seem to always win, some also draw the short stick. You need to know how to be a good sport and not a sore loser. There will be other days. And besides, it's only a game. *The 18th is encouraging.* **◖** *Finish what you've started when the moon rises late.*

Υ ⓩ

reSIStance. You need to take care of yourself. For in this world of pestilence, disease, parasites, viruses, and M.B.A.s, there are many threats to your well-being. You need to ward off that which invades the body, but also those who would rob the soul. Hold up your cross. *The 19th is a good day to make a breakthrough.* **◖** *As the fading moon wanes through the night and into day, take heart . . . and courage.*

⋏ ⓩ

reSIStance reversed. You desperately need to believe. For in this world where there is weakness of body, mind, <u>and</u> spirit—few will find all three strong at once. You need to make "a choice that in choosing offers no choice."[3] *On the 20th, you get your wake-up call.* **◖** *When the waning moon rises late in the night, the answer will come . . . as a dream within a dream.*

⌁ Ⓢ

Sun & Stars. You need to see how you fit into the larger picture. For in this Universe of seemingly random events and huge distances, everything somehow goes together. You need to connect the dots. You need to put the pieces of the puzzle into place. *The 21st is a good day to make the connection.* **◖** *When the Quarter Moon sets in the dawn's early light, hear the bugle, salute, and repeat your pledge.*

---

[3] Sherlock Holmes, upon reading the palm of a young woman on the moors. Pinewood Studios production of Sir Arthur Conan Doyle's *Hound of the Baskervilles*.

↑ Ⓣ

Triumph. Tuesday's child, it's said, is full of grace and, therefore, never falls upon its face—except, of course, in the line of duty. When the summons comes, you must answer the call. For it is your duty we are discussing here. *On Tuesday you will get your marching orders.* ◖*Watch for the Egg Moon in morning. Then make your move.*

↓ Ⓘ

Triumph reversed. You need to come back fighting. For in this world of conflict and competing interests, there are more losers than winners. Not everyone can be on top. If you cannot lead, follow up the rear. But first choose sides. *Mark the 22nd down.* ◖ *When you see the Quarter Moon rising, it's time to hit the showers.*

▶ Ⓑ

Birth. Though the day you were born is a mystery to me, this much is sure and clear: It's a day that you know by heart and two others will never forget. You need to honor your parents, if not also accept them. *By your next birthday, you will get your wish.* ◖*When you waken to a Quarter Moon, go back to sleep and dream your wish.*

◀ Ⓖ

Birth reversed. You need to evolve. For in this world of ours, things are changing by the minute—and so are you. You need to crawl before you stand and walk. You need to gurgle before you talk. And you need to go through a gawky stage before you shed your baby fat. *Mark the 23rd in red.* ◖ *As the Quarter Moon begins its gentle wane, start tying up loose ends.*

M Ⓔ

fEmale. You need to trust your sixth sense. For in this world of icons, dialogue boxes, and double clicks of the computer mouse, you can't find your way around unless you hunt and peck. You need to get out on the networks and do some hunting and gathering. *The 24th provides you with a choice.* ◖ *As the moon starts to show its horns again, you sharpen yours.*

Ⴟ Ⲉ

f**E**male reversed. You need to get in touch with your male side. For in this world where a strong body is thought to be a healthy mind— and where the men smell sweet—you need to pump some iron if you want to compete. *Set aside the 25th for lifting weights.* Ⲉ *As the moon begins to waste away, honor the one who taught you everything.*

Ⲙ Ⲙ

Male. Monday's child, they say, is blessed with fairness of the face, eyes deep with truth and set with trust. For eye to eye the look is passed between men of equal faith . . . in themselves. You need not speak to make your point. Among buddies, it is all understood. *By Monday, things will be old hat.* Ⲉ *As the waning moon leaves behind the dead of night, come out like the deer in the daylight.*

Ⲙ Ⲱ

Male reversed. You need to get in touch with your female side. For in this slick-backed world of ours, you can't get the look without a blow dryer. Take a look in the mirror, fella. When's the last time you shaved? And those old jeans just don't cut it anymore. *The 26th is a day for seeing the truth.* Ⲉ *When the thin moon rises just before the sun, things will have their last hoorah.*

ↆ Ⲉ

Love. You need to have a companion. For in this world of ours, things are inclined to pair up. You need your parents, sisters, broth- ers, cousins, aunts, and uncles. You need your friend, lover, partner, mate, or pet. You need your peers, colleagues, cronies, and cohorts. You need the social contact. *Are you free on the 27th?* Ⲉ *Beware the Dark of the Moon. The currents of love run dark and deep.*

ↆ Ⲉ

Love reversed. You need your privacy. For in this overpopulated world of ours, the roar, race, and rush of the crowd can be madding.

You need some time to yourself. You need to have some space. You need to be happily left alone. *The 28th will offer peace and quiet.* Ⓒ *As the moon retreats into itself, so should you.*

� ⊗

be**ING**. You need to discover your passion. For in this procreative Universe of ours, there are many ways and means of expression. Only you can unlock the secrets of yours. You need to discover what turns you on. You need to get your creative juices flowing. *Set the date for the 29th.* Ⓒ *When in the dawn scant moon you see, get thee to a nunnery.*

✿ Ⓒ

h**O**me. Sunday's child—the old rhyme goes—is glad to put on dress-up clothes, wear smiles from ear to ear, and go to church. You need nothing more than a wing and a prayer. Godspeed. *By Sunday, you will know the parable of the week.* Ⓒ *When the old moon goes, so does its pull on you. Now is the time to get ready to push.*

� Ⓒ

h**O**me reversed. Saturday's child—the saying goes—has a way of roaming down the road. The far, wide journey of a single lifetime knows not the end, yet makes its way there regardless. You need to follow your path to where it leads. *On Saturday you can always sleep in.* Ⓒ *When the final Crescent Moon rises with the sun, wake to a stirring in your soul.*

⋈ Ⓒ Ⓒ

Destiny. You need to achieve your own purpose. For in this Universe of ours, every planet, every moon, and every sun is unique. You need to make your own way along the course that has been set for you. You need to work with your fate in order to make your own destiny. *At the outside, it will be by the 30th.* Ⓒ *When the sun and moon align—and the moon is new again—mark the waterline. Watch for a solar eclipse.*

◘

weird. You need to stand apart from the crowd. For in this world where most things operate on the average, there is a wide range; and it is the extremes that create the curve. You need to set the pace. You need to check and counterbalance. *You will see what it all amounts to by the end of the month.* ◙ *When day or night, there is no moon to see, prepare to start anew.*

EXTRA CREDIT

To determine the right time of the month. Mix up your Runes while you think of your question: **When's the right day to _____?** ask for a raise? pop the question? send in my application? buy a lottery ticket? Reach into your Runes and grab the one that feels right. Then, look up your Rune (upright or reversed) in this Reading's Answer section. Consult the *italic* portion of the text. You're going to be getting two answers. One is a calendar date, and the other is a lunar date. You'll have to decide which makes more sense. To find out when the moon will be in the phase described, consult your wall calendar, almanac, or newspaper.

EXTRA, EXTRA CREDIT!

To make Moon Stones. Get yourself five squares of paper, five matchsticks, or five similar stones and draw a moon on each, like this:

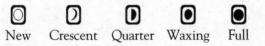

New   Crescent   Quarter   Waxing   Full

Put your Moon Stones in your hands and ask, **When will such and such happen?** When will I know about this or that? Or **When will the moon be right for _____?** Then draw one stone. Look at the shape of the moon. Check your wall calendar, newspaper, or almanac to see when the moon will next be in the phase you have drawn. That's the luckiest time.

But take care! If your moon Rune turns up reversed, it stands for the opposite phase. A Crescent Moon that is upside down (🌑) stands for the final crescent phase. A Quarter Moon upside down (🌑) is the Third Quarter. A waxing moon that is reversed (🌑) is a waning moon.

You can also look up your moon phase in this Reading's Tools section to find the Rune that goes with it. Look up your Rune in the answers and read the *italic* portion of the text.

Go on to the next Reading whenever you are ready to continue.

Reading #11

WHAT WAS I BORN TO BE?
(Give me the powers)

In this Reading you will use your Zodiac sign to receive your Runic horoscope. You can also use this Reading to draw or cast Runes in order to learn what talents, skills, and powers you will need in the days ahead.

I I I

RUNE TOOLS

Here is how the Runes match up with the Zodiac signs you know and love . . .

BIRTH DATE[1]	ZODIAC SIGN	RUNES
March 21 to April 20	Aries	ᚠ ᚢ
April 21 to May 21	Taurus	ᚦ ᚠ
May 22 to June 21	Gemini	ᚱ ᚲ
June 22 to July 22	Cancer	ᚷ ᚹ

---

[1] Starting and ending dates for each sign are approximate. If you generally use another system to compute your sign, go right ahead.

BIRTH DATE	ZODIAC SIGN	RUNES	
July 23 to August 22	Leo	ᚺ	ᚾ
August 23 to September 22	Virgo	ᛁ	ᛃ
September 23 to October 22	Libra	ᛇ	ᛈ
October 23 to November 22	Scorpio	ᛉ	ᛊ
November 23 to December 21	Sagittarius	ᛏ	ᛒ
December 22 to January 20	Capricorn	ᛖ	ᛗ
January 21 to February 19	Aquarius	ᛚ	ᛜ
February 20 to March 20	Pisces	ᛟ	ᛞ
□	Don't Know		

HOW TO

To find your Runic horoscope . . .

1. Just look up your date of birth or Zodiac sign in the previous chart. You can also look up the dates of family members and friends.

2. Jot down the two Runes that match up with your sign.

Scratch Pad

Jot down your Runes here.

⧇ Look up your Runes in this Reading's Answer section.

THE ANSWERS

The answers appear in the traditional order of the Runes, but they are listed in pairs. Reversed Runes immediately follow their upright counterparts (**ᚷ, ᚺ, ᛏ, ᛁ, ᛜ, ᛃ, ᛋ, ᛈ, ᛗ**, and **ᛟ** have no reversals).

F U Th A R K G W H N I Y Ê P Z S T B E M L X O D ⟨⟩

ᚠ ᚢ ᚦ ᚨ ᚱ ᚲ ᚷ ᚹ ᚺ ᛏ ᛁ ᛜ ᛃ ᚲ ᛇ ᛋ ᛏ ᛒ ᛖ ᛗ ᛚ ᛜ ᛟ ᛞ ⟨⟩

K=C & Q; W=V; Y=J

ᚠ ⒡ ᚢ ⒰

Fortune and l**U**ck. Well, Aries, you know who you are, so what more can I say? Your Runes are the cow (**Fehu**) <u>and</u> the bull (**Uruz**). You are the Ram of the Zodiac. To put it gently, you make beautiful

music as fast and furiously as you can. You are creative, fertile, prolific—and as quick as a jackrabbit—at whatever you do. From your
ranks come a surprising number of folk heroes and living legends.[2]
It seems like anyone who can speak for the rest of us has a chance
at center stage. You were born to the breed. For even if you don't
walk around trying to save the world, you give others something to
emulate. If you can make your point in a couple of sound bites—a
hundred words or less—you will forge ahead. Whatever you do, do
it with conviction. With both fortune and luck on your side, you
should have little difficulty in achieving what you want once you
decide what it is. Your powers are these . . .

F Ⓕ *Creative energy—You have the power to build bridges, construct
buildings, genetically reengineer the crops, and increase profits in the
process. But before you can develop, you may have to tear something
down.*

ᛃ Ⓙ *Destructive energy—You have the power to bulldoze forests,
upturn the earth, downsize the workforce, and bully others. But it only
works in the short term. Demolish with care.*

U Ⓤ *Force—You have the power to take the cow by the horns, the dog
by the scruff, and the bull by the . . . ring in his nose. But those who do
not trust in luck will seldom know it. Do you believe?*

ᚾ Ⓝ *Counterforce—You have the power to line up your ducks, put up
your dukes, and stick to your guns. In order to improve your luck, avoid
the ones who rip you off, lure you with candy, or try to trick you. But
don't be paranoid either.*

ᚦ Ⓣⱶ **ᚠ** Ⓐ

faiTH and fAte. So, Taurus, how long have you had these bold, new
ideas? As the Bull of the Zodiac, it would seem you aspire to influence as many as you can get to. Can it be sheer coincidence that

---

[2] Douglas MacArthur, Janis Joplin, and Steve McQueen all had Aries rising.
Bach, Brando, and Charlemagne all had the sun in Aries. And JFK had his
moon in Aries.

your part of the Zodiac is overpopulated with leading figures—like RFK, Jackie O, and Valentino?[3] Since your Runes are the thorn (**Thurisaz**) <u>and</u> the mouth (**Ansuz**), it would appear you are good at making your keen words work for you. With fate on your side, and faith in your camp, the signs look good for a clean sweep in at least your native state. Remember, though, true power is not in knowing how to get to the top, it's in doing the <u>right</u> thing once you get there. For starters, you might as well come forth, take the soapbox, and give us your best pitch. Just remember, these days, it's mostly done with smoke and mirrors. All power to you. Once you gain the upper hand over us, please try to be gentle. Your powers are these . . .

ᚦ *Divine right—Within your borders, you have the power to set the rules, call the shots, defend the faith, conduct public works projects, and collect taxes. But without a steady revenue stream, you won't have a throne to sit on, let alone a pot to . . . spit in.*

ᚢ *Divine intervention—You have the power to assemble peacefully, state your opinion openly, petition in writing, be secure in your house, and (for the time being) own arms. But without the support of the courts, you will soon be defenseless. Hang on to your ammunition.*

ᚨ *God willing—You have the power to do the best that you can, and even more sometimes, weather permitting and God on your side. But in order to return the favor, you must remain true to your word.*

ᚢ *God wanting—You have the power to crawl out from under the worst conditions, even if it's the act of an angry god. In order to incur a favor, you may have to do penance. Watch your cursing.*

ᚱ **ᚲ**

Reality and **Karma**. Gemini, Gemini, what can I say? You are destined to go in two different ways . . . play two different roles . . . wear

---

[3] Robert Kennedy had Taurus rising, Jacqueline Kennedy Onassis had her moon in Taurus, and Valentino had the sun in Taurus.

two different hats . . . put on two different masks. Your sign represents the Twins of the Zodiac. But are you Tragedy or Comedy today? It comes as no surprise that your sign has influenced a great many theatrical personalities.[4] So if the smell of greasepaint appeals to you, I guess you were born to the breed. Your Runes—Raidho (the journey) and Kenaz (the light)—indicate that you will surely take your show on the road. But first you will have to get your act together. One among you said, "All the world's a stage."[5] And you will surely make your living on it. Know, though, it takes a great deal of energy to put up a false front. And it takes not only talent but practice to be convincing. Under the influence of both Reality and Karma, you will need to suspend your own disbelief in order to find your true motivation. At any rate, choose your parts well. It is your job to help the rest of us understand our own humanity, and we could all use a tear or two as well as a couple of laughs. Your powers are these . . .

R **ℝ** *Real Time*—*You have the power to witness what is taking place, to follow the linear sequence of events, observe, participate, and take notes. To understand completely, you sort of have to be there.*

Y **ⓨ** *Virtual Reality*—*You have the power to create your own reality, live in your own fantasy world, and explore your imaginary kingdoms in 3-D. But until you interact with the real thing, you will only know illusion.*

< **ⓒ** *"Good" Karma*—*You have the power to make a difference . . . to say something worth saying, to do something worth doing, to make something worth making, and to sacrifice something worth giving. The higher the price, the greater the reward.*

> **ⓞ** *"Bad" Karma*—*You have the power to make the lives of others a tolerable human experience or a lesson in mental cruelty. Just bear in mind, it all comes back in time.*

---

[4] Hope, Diller, Astaire, and Garbo all had Gemini rising. Isadora Duncan had the sun in Gemini. And Jack Benny, Bette Davis, Joanne Woodward, and Shirley Temple all had the moon in Gemini.
[5] Shakespeare had Neptune in Gemini.

ᚷ Ⓖ ᚠ Ⓥ Ⓦ

Gifts and Wonder. Well, Cancer, what can I say to the gifted? Pure and simply, you are a work of art. Is it any wonder that Rembrandt, Dali, and Picasso are among you?[6] They showed the rest of us how good it could be. You were born to the breed. Your Runes are Gebo (the gift) and Wunjo (joy). With these alone, one could well get through a single lifetime and never wish for more. True to the sign of the Crab, you may be hard on the surface, but soft and sensitive in the core. As you pursue your art, keep your sense of humor, and try not to get hurt. Every now and again, you will have to come out of your shell and grow a new one. In this way alone you bring new form, shape, and substance into the world. But most of all it is your power to interpret life that appeals so much to us. You challenge us to think. We stand before your work with our heads tilted to one side. We can hardly wait to see what you will do next. But just remember, in your search for truth, look also for beauty. And try not to shock our sensitivities too much. Your powers are these . . .

ᚷ Ⓖ Ⓖ *Blessings—You have the power to paint what you see, say what you know, and sing what you feel. But you may have to take a few lessons to master the technique. And you may have to suffer a bit.*

ᚠ Ⓥ Ⓦ *Positive Influence—You have the power to look on the bright side and paint a rosy picture of the world. But unless there is also a pang of pathos, the critics will never buy it.*

ᚲ Ⓐ Ⓦ *Negative Influence—You have the power to cast things in a dim light and paint a bleak picture of the world. But unless there is a ray of hope at the end, the public will snub it.*

ᚺ Ⓗ ᛏ Ⓝ

Hail and Need. So, Leo, who does your hair? Who takes the thorn from your foot? And who cleans up after you? As the Lion of the Zodiac, you know you're the King of the Beasts, so you might as well

---

[6] Rembrandt had the sun in Cancer, Dali had Cancer rising, and Picasso had the moon in Cancer.

roar. From your sign come a remarkable number of big-time entertainers.[7] So I guess you will have to do things larger than life. With the stormy Runes of Hail (**H**agaluz) and Need (**N**audhiz) creating a regular fireworks display of special effects, it should never be a dull moment. You wave your arm, say a few magic words, and produce a white rabbit from your hat. How did you do that? (I guess you were born to the breed!) Heads turn when you make an entrance. The crowd gasps as you execute a sleight of hand. Were it not for you, there would be no spectaculars. All you have to do is find your gimmick, and we'll all be clamoring for more. I'm rooting for you. But just remember, once you've got the Greatest Show on Earth, try not to charge the rest of us too much for general admission. Your powers are these . . .

H Ⓗ *Static electricity—You have the power to get yourself charged up, electrified, magnetized, and psyched. You have the power to thrill, shock, and jolt the living daylights out of us. Better watch your own voltmeter. Check your pulse.*

⧈ Ⓝ *Nuclear energy—You have the power to crack things apart and figure out how they work. And you have the power to fuse things back together. Manage your limited resources wisely. Recharge your battery from time to time. And turn off a few lights.*

Ⅰ Ⓘ **⬦** Ⓨ Ⓙ

Ice and Year. So, Virgo, what's your secret? As the Virgin of the Zodiac, you must have a few—or at the very least, an idiosyncrasy or two? Or one skeleton neatly tucked away in the back of your closet? They are inclined to call you "neat," "fastidious," and orderly to a fault. So I guess it's no wonder that an incredible number of eccentrics have a strong Virgo in their charts.[8] What can I say? You were born to the breed. Feisty, often quaint, and all in all downright interesting, you are a <u>real</u> character. Your Runes are Isa (river of ice) and Jera (the harvest), and as a result, you can go from one season

[7] Both P. T. Barnum and Cecil B. De Mille had Leo rising in their charts. Mick Jagger has the sun in Leo. And Streisand has the moon.
[8] The reclusive Howard Hughes had Virgo rising, as did the self-indulgent child prodigy Mozart. Elizabeth I, the Virgin Queen, had the sun in Virgo.

to another overnight. The rest of us wonder a bit about you sometimes. But for the most part we find your compulsive ways charming. And we like the results only you can deliver quite so matter-of-factly. You make it look so easy. Just be careful not to violate your own standards—or worse yet, get caught. We like our Virgins to be the real thing. You wouldn't want to disappoint us. Your powers are these . . .

❙ Ⓤ *Inertia—You have the power to store up your energy, put on a layer of winter fat, and prepare to hibernate. But just as easily you can drain yourself, burn off weight, or emerge to see your shadow. What makes rocks in the desert roll? Gather no moss.*

❖ Ⓨ Ⓐ Ⓤ ⓡ *Momentum—You have the power to take a running leap, a flying jump, and maybe even a double back flip. Just be sure to pick up enough speed before you make the attempt. And if at first you don't succeed, the third time is always the charm.*

♪ ⓪ Ⓚ Ⓟ

h**E**lp and ho**P**e. Well, Libra, it seems as if the scales are tipped in your favor, at least when it comes to running for office. There are an incredible number of politicians with Libra strongly in their charts.[9] Your Runes are **E**ihwaz (the yew) and **P**erthro (the dice cup). So it's clear that to play this game you must be willing to bend in the wind and take a risk or two during the campaign. With help and hope on your side, the odds would seem to be even. (But you would never be satisfied with a draw.) As you prepare for this life, be careful that your business dealings are all aboveboard. If you ever smoke anything, don't inhale. And be careful whom you sleep with. We like our public figures to behave better than we do. Once you get to high office, don't forget who voted for you. Your powers are these . . .

♪ Ⓔ Ⓔ *Defensive Moves—You have the power to outsmart, outwit, outmaneuver, and outdebate your would-be opponents. But you may*

---

[9] Canada's Trudeau is a sun-sign Libra. John Glenn and Eleanor Roosevelt have the moon in Libra. And England's George VI had Libra rising.

have to do some fancy footwork to avoid the mud being slung. Duck behind your cleanest laundry. Careful not to get tangled in the lines.

ᚲ ⟨ᛈ⟩ *Rune for Office—You have the power to throw your hat in the ring and announce your ambitions to the world. That only takes confidence. Now comes the hard part. You must also be convincing. Better hang on to your day job until you get the cushy one.*

ᛉ ⟨ᛩ⟩ *Rune out of Office—You have the power to concede the race at any point along the way. But you never know until the final ballot is cast. And who can tell? You may yet come out of nowhere to win as the dark horse.*

ᛏ ⟨ᛉ⟩ ᛊ ⟨ᛊ⟩

reSIStance and Stars. Say, Scorpio, is it true what they say about you? Is your bite half as good as your sting? Or once you've mesmerized us, are we just too eager to know the difference? Among your ranks are an inordinate number of saints and sinners—and sometimes it's difficult to tell which is which.[10] Either way, you beguile us so, it seems we simply can't resist. But a Scorpion for a Zodiac sign? (Next thing you'll be wanting a tattoo.) Your Runes are Elhaz (the antlers of the elk) and Sowilo (the rays of the sun). The two, together, arm you well and keep you warm. They also tend to draw attention and invite conflict. But isn't that just what you hoped to attract? We see in your eyes a look we both respect and fear. Once you have us locked spellbound in your grip, it could go any which way you choose. But mercy . . . that only adds to the excitement. Your powers are these . . .

ᛏ ⟨ᛉ⟩ *Body chemistry—You have the power to attract others with your scent. And if Mother Nature hasn't been good to you, there's always Armani, Yves Saint Laurent, and Shalimar. There are ways to make heads turn, you know.*

---

[10] Castro and Elvis have Scorpio rising. The radical Trotsky and the heretical Martin Luther had the sun in Scorpio. Billy Graham and Charles Manson both have Scorpio in the Eighth House.

🏹 Ⓩ *Alchemy—You have the power to weave your love charm with yohimbé bark, ginseng root, garlic, or whatever turns you on. But love won falsely is the shortest kind. And this kind of magic can be undone.*

🗡 Ⓢ *Solar Energy—You have the power to aim toward the light, soak up the sun, and watch your skin change color like a chameleon. But the surgeon general has determined you shouldn't worship the sun—so even this in moderation.*

⬆ Ⓣ ⮞ Ⓑ

Triumph and **B**irth. Well, Sagittarius, I don't have to tell you how to put on a good show. Among your ranks come a surprising number of performing artists.[11] As the half-horse, half-man of the Zodiac, one would expect you'd be a regular satyr! But your passions tend to run on the titillating rather than the blatant side. Your Runes are **T**iwaz (the warrior) and **B**erkano (the birches), which imply that glory comes from persistence. With triumph a distinct possibility in your life, and the experience of birth (or rebirth) noted, you stand to leave your mark on the world through your dedicated labor. Whatever you choose to do for a living, your inimitable style is your own, and cannot be readily copied. You are simply one who stands out from the rest. You are your own genius. And we admire you for that. But what we like most of all is when you dazzle us. Your powers are these . . .

⬆ Ⓣ *Strike Force—You have the power to overwhelm, outgun, and outcharm those who would oppose or resist you. But you will also want to have a contingency plan, in case things—as they are inclined to do—go wrong. It's just Murphy's Law.*

⬇ Ⓛ *Counteroffensive—You have the power to reconnoiter, reposition, or realign. You can even retreat. These tactics are most effective if they contain an element of surprise. Do something we'd never think of.*

---

[11] Famous stripper Gypsy Rose Lee had Sagittarius rising (along with the audience). Guitarist Jimi Hendrix had the sun in Sagittarius. And Beethoven, Brahms, and Liszt all had the moon in Sagittarius.

ᛒ Ⓑ *Labor*—You have the power to put your back into each shovelful you sling. But remember to bend at the knees. And don't forget your breathing.

ᛇ ⑨ *Delivery*—You have the power to expand and contract, flex and release, lift and separate. But you may have to bite the bullet in the process. Try not to get bent out of shape.

ᛗ Ⓔ ᛗ Ⓜ

fEmale and Male. Well, Capricorn, we all know how conservative you are supposed to be . . . straitlaced and traditional. So why are there so many controversial figures who share your sign?[12] I guess it takes a conservative to get enough power to be a good revolutionary. You were born to the breed. Your Runes are Ehwaz (the horse) and Mannaz (the man). Combined with the goat, it makes for quite a menagerie. You are skilled at exerting your influence on the world by taking a firm stand. You stretch to the limits of your tether. You champ at the bit. You resent the reins. But we like you because you know how to lead us in the right direction. For the best effect, balance out your aggressive male tendencies with a woman's sensitivity. To get our attention, you will want to speak in your most authoritative voice. But whatever you do, don't betray our trust. Your powers are these . . .

ᛗ Ⓔ *Female Energy*—You have the power to express yourself in a firm but unthreatening way. Your best weapons are motherhood, apple pie, and womanly wiles. There are three ways, after all, to reach our hearts and touch our souls.

ᛗ ③ *Male Energy*—You have the power to raise your voice, wrinkle your brow, and act like you really mean it (this time). But remember, some find it is easier to ask forgiveness than permission. What you don't want to know, don't ask.

[12] Darwin had Capricorn rising, as well as the moon. Mao, Nixon, Capone, and Martin Luther King had the sun in Capricorn. And mystic to the Tsar of Russia, Rasputin, had the moon.

ᛗ Ⓜ *Male Energy*—You have the power to be fairly aggressive, at least with a pair of hedge clippers and a lawn mower. And if left to your own devices, who knows how far you'd encroach on your neighbor's yard? In staking out your claims, it's best to leave easements.

ᛉ Ⓦ *Female Energy*—You have the power to share the responsibility, to split the tasks, and to divide the chores. It will all come easier if everyone takes a turn, but someone will have to be the leader. (Isn't it your turn tonight?)

ᚠ Ⓛ **ᛜ** ⓧ

Love and beING. Well, Aquarius, they say it is the dawning of your age. And I certainly hope it is. For there are an alarming number of philosophers who share your sun sign, or who have the sun rising in Aquarius, or the moon.[13] You were born to the breed. So say something profound for us. Or at least give us a kiss. Your Runes are Laguz (the water) and Ingwaz (the love goddess). There can be no other conclusion . . . the waters of passion flow through your veins . . . the waters of life pulse in your wrist (and other body parts). As the Water Bearer of the Zodiac, you are connected to the Eternal Stream. And when you speak, it's as if you are channeling higher thoughts. With both love and sex in your Runes, it looks like it will not be <u>all</u> work for you. It's okay to be sensuous. Despite your bravado and libido, the rest of us see in you the truth we all aspire to. You speak to our highest hopes and best ideals. But beware. Some will use your own words against you. Your powers are these . . .

ᚠ Ⓛ *Love*—You have the power to give a damn about others, a damn about what's going on in the world, and a damn about what's going to happen tomorrow. But in your rush to save humanity, don't forget your best friend.

---

[13] Jefferson and Marx had Aquarius rising. Dickens, Lincoln, and FDR had the sun in Aquarius. And both Lenin and John Lennon had the moon, along with Yeats, Voltaire, and Sandburg.

↙ ⏢ *Hatred*—*You have the power to turn your back on the world and not give a damn about what they do in Washington, London, Moscow, Tokyo, or Berlin. You have the power to shut people out of your life—but that will only shut you in.*

�֍ ⏴ *Orgasm*—*You have the power to let loose with the biggest bang in the Universe. You have the power to create new life and assure the survival of the species, while—at the same time—enjoying yourself. It's not such a bad lot, self-indulgence.*

✖ ⏢ ⋈ ⏴

hOme and Destiny. Well, Pisces, what a great idea you've had—and now if you can just express it in your own inimitable way, we'll give you a standing ovation. This comes as no surprise, I guess, since among your ranks are geniuses by the score. Composers, singers, scientists, dancers . . . even Einstein himself.[14] You were born to the breed. But genius is a solitary business. Your Runes are Othala (the homeland) and Dagaz (the day), which indicates the things you like the best are those you choose to do on your own time. For despite the two fishes in your Zodiac sign, you are a solo artist—after all. With all your admirers flocking around you, how can you find the time to do your work? Your life is full of the music of the spheres. It is the music of life in progress . . . sometimes flat and sometimes sharp . . . sometimes the blues, and sometimes hip-hop. It's a nice tune to tap your foot to. I give it a 99. Your powers are these . . .

✖ ⏢ *Introversion*—*You have the power to come home at the end of the day and shut out the noise and confusion of the rest of the world. You have the power to find the silence inside you, where your beauty dwells.*

✖ ⏢ *Extroversion*—*You have the power to get out and be with people. And even if you have to sit in different sections of the restaurant, you can still look at each other across the partitions. Pass the salt, will ya?*

---

[14] Einstein had the sun in Pisces, as did Caruso, Chopin, and Nureyev. And with the moon in Pisces: Helen Keller, Michelangelo, and Shelley. Hitchcock had Pisces rising.

▣ ⊡ ⊡ *Continuity—You have the power to make your story unfold as if it were a logical sequence of events. You have the power to put the puzzle together, and find the bigger picture that the pieces make.*

⊡

weird. If you're not sure exactly when you were born, that's weird indeed. But what the hay. Take as your sign the one that's never talked about in the Zodiac, old Ophiuchus the Serpent Holder himself, the great doctor of the heavens, blessed with the power to heal all mortal aches and pains. And if you can't be one, marry one. Your power is limited to just the one (but some say it is everything) . . .

⊡ *Medicine—You have the power to diagnose the illness, treat the symptoms, and get the good drugs. But don't forget it's mostly bedside manner. Physician, heal thyself.*[15]

EXTRA CREDIT

To identify your powers. Mix up your Runes while you think of your question: **What strengths will I need to call upon in order to _____?** What powers will I need in the months ahead? Or—for an interesting revelation—simply **Give me the powers.**

Reach into your Runes and select the three that feel attracted to your hand. Or toss a handful of Runes on the ground and draw three. Note whether your Runes are upright or reversed. Then find them in this Reading's Answer section. Read the *italic* portion of the text.

Each of your Runes will tell you one skill, or power, that you can draw upon. It generally takes a combination of tools to get a single job done. So if you think you need more than three Runes, draw, draw again.

[15] Luke 4:23

EXTRA, EXTRA CREDIT!

Maybe, maybe not. Using the Yes/No Rune you made in the Extra, Extra Credit section of Reading #1, you can add new dimension to your yes/no Readings by considering what reversals mean. Just ask your yes/no question as before and toss your Rune. Look at it and note whether it is upright (😳 🆖) or reversed (🆘 🔛). Interpret a reversed YES as "maybe not." Interpret a reversed NO as "maybe." If the answer is not what you'd hoped, you always have the opportunity to work on it some more.

Go on to the next Reading whenever you are ready to continue.

Reading #12

WHAT AM I BECOMING?
(Tell me the skinny)

___

In this Reading, you will be using your Runes like a timepiece to find out what stage of your life you're going through and what changes you can expect this year. Or you can also use this Reading to draw or cast Runes to learn what qualities become you now and what tools you need.

<7<7<7

RUNE TOOLS

Every Rune has a number, as well as a sound and a name. The number is simply the Rune's order in the Futhark sequence.

1	ᚠ	7	ᚷ	13	ᛃ	19	ᛗ
2	ᚢ	8	ᚹ	14	ᛈ	20	ᛉ
3	ᚦ	9	ᚺ	15	ᛉ	21	ᛚ
4	ᚨ	10	ᚾ	16	ᛊ	22	ᛜ
5	ᚱ	11	ᛁ	17	ᛏ	23	ᛟ
6	ᚲ	12	ᛇ	18	ᛒ	24	ᛞ
						25	☐

In ABC's . . .

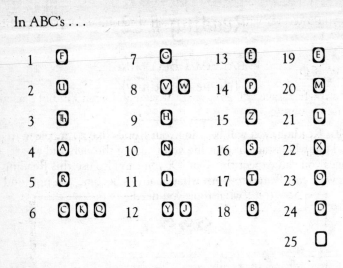

1	Ⓕ	7	Ⓖ	13	Ⓔ̂	19	Ⓔ
2	Ⓤ	8	ⓋⓌ	14	Ⓟ	20	Ⓜ
3	Ⓣh	9	Ⓗ	15	Ⓩ	21	Ⓛ
4	Ⓐ	10	Ⓝ	16	Ⓢ	22	Ⓧ
5	Ⓡ	11	Ⓘ	17	Ⓣ	23	Ⓞ
6	ⓒⓀⓆ	12	ⓎⒿ	18	Ⓑ	24	Ⓓ
						25	⬜

Since there are 24 Runes in all (not counting Blank), they can be neatly divided into two sets of 12. Naturally, the Runes in the first half can be matched up, one for one, with the Runes in the second half—to form 12 pairs. The pairs are (reading from the top down, ᚠ and ᛁ, ᚢ and ᚴ, ᚦ and ᛏ . . .):

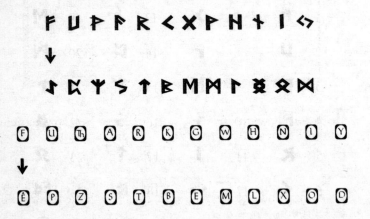

So far so good, right? But the really fascinating thing is, each pair of Runes makes sense together. This Reading's Answer section will help you interpret what the pairs mean when linked to your age in years.

HOW TO

To learn what stage you are going through and what kind of person you are becoming . . .

1   Just jot down your current age on the Scratch Pad. Also jot down the ages of others you care to ask about.

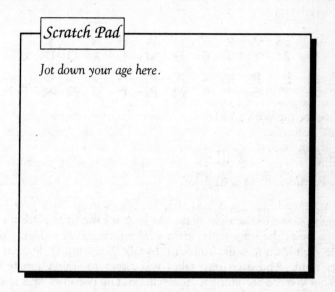

Scratch Pad

Jot down your age here.

2   If you are under 26 (you lucky duck), just look up your number in this Reading's Answer section.

3   For those over 25, there's a trick . . .

■   If you are between 26 and 50, first subtract 25 from your age, and look up the resulting number in the Answer section.

■   If you are 51 to 75, subtract 50. Then look up the total in the Answer section.

■ For those over 75, subtract 75, then look up the total in the Answer section. And, for the benefit of my Old Grandma, if you are over 100, subtract 100 first.[1]

THE ANSWERS

The answers appear in the traditional order of the Runes, but they are listed in pairs. Reversed Runes immediately follow their upright counterparts (✕, ᚺ, ✝, ᛁ, ◇, ↑, ⊱, ✦, ᛉ, and ☐ have no reversals).

F	U	Th	A	R	K	G	W	H	N	I	Y
Ê	P	Z	S	T	B	E	M	L	X	O	D	O

K=C & Q; W=V; Y=J

ᚠ Ⓕ   ↑ Ⓔ

1. Fortune.   **13.** hElp

If you are 1, 13, 26, 38, 51, 63, 76, 88, or even (holy cow!) 101, you've come to the right place. At least it's the right place for you. You are at the stage when great strides forward are suddenly possible. You learn to walk. You learn to talk. You learn to do what others want. And each step takes you closer to your ultimate goal. What you are becoming is: Yourself. And no one else. This is a year for taking a big step forward in the process. But you might have to take two steps backwards first. Years of transition can be like that. So call on your resources. Gather your defenses. And don't be afraid to ask for help. You have these things going for you . . .

[1] This numerological method is based loosely on a technique developed by Roland Dionys Jossé and presented in *Die Tala der Raunen* (1955). Thanks to Edred Thorsson for describing it in *Rune Might* (1989). *Runes in Ten Minutes* uses 25 Runes instead of Jossé's 16. So instead of dividing by 16s, we subtract by 25s to get the same effect.

Ϝ Ⓕ *Body.* You are fortunate at having been born with however many fingers, toes, and other appendages you ended up with. Now let's use them to count off your accomplishments. Your strength comes from controlling your weaknesses.

ϟ Ⓔ *Mind.* You are also fortunate at having the good sense to know when to quit. It is good you are able to see cause and effect. Good, too, that you are able to make decisions based on feedback. You make use of both sense and reason.

ϟ Ⓔ Ⓔ *Spirit.* You are thrice fortunate in knowing how to tell right from wrong, good from bad, and plus from minus. Feelings count just as much as facts in the scheme of things. Listen to the voices in your head. Pay attention to your dreams. And don't forget to say your heartfelt prayers.

Ʋ Ⓤ   **Ϻ** Ⓟ

2. lUck   **14. hoPe**

If you are 2, 14, 27, 39, 52, 64, 77, 89, or (jumpin' Jehoshaphat!) 102, you've found the right place. You are at the stage when it's time to take one giant step forward. And so what if you risk falling flat on your face? Nothing ventured, nothing gained. And sometimes it seems as if you can do no wrong. But other times—well—so what if they laugh at you? It's only at first. In the process of living and learning, what you are becoming is: A Real Human Being. It does you good to try your luck. It does you good to hold out hope. And this is the year, my friend, for doing both. You would seem to be on a roll. You have these things going for you . . .

Ʋ Ⓤ *Charms.* You are lucky to be in your own two shoes. And it's true. You have many things going for you. And many things have come to you on just your pretty smile alone . . . not to mention those sweet-talking lips.

Ⴖ Ⓝ *Amulets.* Whether you hang your horseshoe right side up or upside down, it can bring you nothing ill. Even the nails, they say, are lucky. Believe what you will. But tack up your favorite hex sign.

ᛈ (P) *Tokens.* *You have your Susan B. Anthony dollar for your pocket. You have your fuzzy dice for your car. And—if I know you—you even have your lucky bikini. What can I say? Wear it in good faith.*

ᛃ (J) *Talismans.* *You have your medals, emblems, and medallions. You have lucky necklaces and bracelets. But for the best luck of all, carve the entire Futhark on your favorite charm:* ᚠ ᚢ ᚦ ᚨ ᚱ ᚲ ᚷ ᚹ ᚺ ᚾ ᛁ ᛃ ᛇ ᛈ ᛉ ᛊ ᛏ ᛒ ᛖ ᛗ ᛞ ᛚ ᛝ ᛟ ᛞ.

ᚦ (Th) ᛉ (Z)

3. faiTh **15.** reSIStance

If you are 3, 15, 28, 40, 53, 65, 78, 90, or (leapin' lizards!) 103, you've turned to the right place. You are in a stage when it's not only possible to get into serious mischief but it's almost impossible not to. One way or the other, doors open, and you go through them, not always thinking clearly about what you might be walking into. Yet again, there is hardly a choice. This year you get the urge to explore a strange and exciting new world. You turn away the hand that would hold you in check. You ignore the advice of your elders. And you have no interest in reading the warning labels. So, my friend, you will have to fend for yourself this year. There is a moral to be learned now, but it does not necessarily come from a book. Nor can anyone teach it to you. For it is your lesson that needs learning . . . by you. You are becoming a whole new person. I know you are made of the right stuff. You have these things going for you . . .

ᚦ (Th) *Trust.* *There is no shortage of rules to live by, codes to abide, and standards to conform to. You must assume that most will play by the rules—at least, sort of. But don't be naïve. Have confidence mostly in yourself.*

ᚦ (Yl) *Doubt.* *There is no reason to be foolish when it comes to placing your trust in others. You can smell a rotten potato from a couple aisles away, can't you? Let the buyer beware—especially if you're picking up the tab.*

Ψ Ⓩ *Will.* There is a look in your eye. There is a sound in your voice. And there is a way you hold yourself. Let your conviction show through your brave deeds. And whatever you do, don't doubt yourself . . . or look away.

↑ Ⓩ *Wit.* Necessity, they say, is the mother of invention. For where there is a will, there is a way. You can avert many a crisis by making use of diversionary tactics. Nothing says you have to mean every word that you say. It's okay, sometimes, to bluff your way out of a predicament.

Ϝ Ⓐ   **Ϟ** Ⓢ

4. fAte   **16. Sun & Stars**

If you are 4, 16, 29, 41, 54, 66, 79, 91, or (bless your soul!) 104, you're at the right place, and this is the right time. At this phase in your life, you find yourself getting a fresh taste for freedom. Things come together in no uncertain terms this year, even if they fly apart in the process. You get behind the wheel of your own car and drive off to do whatever it is that enchants you. Life's lessons, they say, are sometimes learned the hard way. But all in all, the things that are meant to be reveal themselves to you, especially now. No one but you will ever know it all or understand it completely. The point is, what you are becoming is the Person You Were Born to Be. For just as the sun, moon, stars, and planets have their respective orbits to course, you have yours. And this is Now. What you have going for you is this . . .

Ϝ Ⓐ *Watchwords.* In the beginning was the word . . . and it was all-powerful. So from your dictionary, thesaurus, book of quotations, or Holy Bible, take the key words that will guide you. Adopt a motto. Develop a slogan. And live accordingly.

↓ Ⓥ *Whispers.* From the mouths of babes, they say, come otherwise unspoken truths (which sometimes hurt). Speak not quite as bluntly as the children do in real life. But to your own mirror, confess your inner secrets and accept the truth about yourself in silence.

ϟ Ⓢ *Symbols. The sun comes and goes each day a little farther north or south. The moon comes along each night, a little bigger or smaller and a tad later. And the stars just keep on circling in the sky. Watch these eternal symbols closely.*

Ⓡ ᛦ   **↑ Ⓣ**

5. Reality   17. Triumph

If you are 5, 17, 30, 42, 55, 67, 80, 92, or even (jeez-o-man!) 105, you've found your place in this book. And—don't look now—but here comes a final checkpoint, Charlie . . . and a last chance to prove yourself before moving on. It is an anxious, expectant, and tentative moment. But if you want to get to the other side of the road, you will have to cross. Needless to say, this can be a year of irony or nostalgia. If you want to savor the moment, now's your chance. In the process of gathering your life's experience, you are becoming a Truth-teller. Reach within yourself this year. In the final analysis it doesn't matter what others think, say, or do—as long as you know what the truth is. If you haven't found it yet, keep looking. You have these things going for you . . .

Ⓡ ᛦ *Wheels. Everything that's anything in the Universe turns in a big wide sweep. So even when you think you're standing still, you're moving on. You have no choice, except to quit spinning your wheels.*

ᛨ Ⓨ *Ruts. Your road goes ever on . . . despite rain, sleet, snow, or dark of night. But the lanes are not always clear and free of debris. Lucky you know how to dodge.*

↑ Ⓣ *Arrowheads. You have an arsenal of weapons at your disposal. Carry an arrowhead in your pocket, and you will come to no harm. Inscribe it with a ↑ , and you'll always find your target.*

↓ Ⓘ *Plowshares. You have many tools at your command—not to mention all 25 Runes. And they work as well in peace as in war. Put your weapons down now . . . and turn back to the land you fought to save.*

◀ Ⓒ Ⓚ Ⓠ   ▶ Ⓑ

6. Course,   18. Birth
   Quest,
   Karma

If you are 6, 18, 31, 43, 56, 68, 81, 93, or (O wise one!) 106, you've found your answer. Here it is: You are in a phase when you not only blossom, but come into your full bloom. You've made it! But before you bask too much in this moment of attainment, take a gander ahead. In coming to this point, you now have the opportunity to branch off, turn over a new leaf, or even head off on a new spiritual quest. A door would seem to want to open no sooner than another is closed. And this year, yours is revolving. Where will you go out this time? You are becoming A Person by Choice. Your soul is taking shape. Just keep following your own footsteps, and one day you will reach your heights. You have all these things going for you . . .

◀ Ⓒ Ⓝ Ⓠ *Candles. It is such a small and wavering light the candle makes. And yet it puts you in the mood, all right . . . for all kinds of natural acts. Light a few, and you will see the world in a different (albeit shadowy) light.*

▶ Ⓢ Ⓝ Ⓠ *Incense. There is no flame, and yet the sandalwood burns. Send your prayers up on its swirling trails of smoke. (That is, of course, as long as the FDA approves.) Seek enlightenment.*

▶ Ⓑ *Blood. You are of the flesh. And the flesh, they say, is weak. So be it. Nothing was meant to last forever, not even tooth, nail, and bone. Save first the women and children. Tend to the newborn.*

◀ Ⓦ *Water. You are of the spirit, which like an endless stream runs back to the sea whence it came. Everything is connected to everything else. All you have to do is tap in. Reach into yourself and make the connection.*

✖

7. Gifts   19. fEmale

If you are 7, 19, 32, 44, 57, 69, 82, 94, or (good golly, Miss Molly!) 107, this is the place where you should be . . . and "X" marks the spot. You have come to the point when you must sow a few oats. So dig here, my friend. This is a year for blossoming. It is a time for mixing and matching, folding and blending, racking and stacking. You must give as well as receive. It is a time for letting the urge within you express itself. In the process of projecting your personality, you are becoming A Well-Rounded Person. The key is to be a little psychic. See with a new sight what lies below the surface. Hear, with new ears, what goes unspoken. Pick up on what others are thinking. A mind is a terrible thing to waste. So is a sixth sense. You have all this going for you . . .

✗ Ⓖ Ⓢ *Magic. You have a trick or two up your sleeve. And with a wave of your magic wand—and a well-rehearsed line of patter—you sure can captivate your audience. (But I think it's all done with mirrors.)*

M Ⓔ *Mystique. You have a certain way about you unlike anyone else on this planet. You have your own little secrets, patented techniques, and sensual wiles. Call them up as needed.*

W Ⓔ *Musk. You have a certain scent about you that either really attracts or really repels. Be a little sensitive to the signals you are sending out. They have a way of attracting all kinds.*

ᚠ Ⓥ Ⓦ   **ᛘ Ⓜ**

8. Wonder   20. Male

If you are 8, 20, 33, 45, 58, 70, 83, 95, or (Lordy, Lordy!) 108, you have found your Runes. But more important, you have come to a point in your life when you must reach your own independent conclusions. It is a time for calling to task all the learning and experience you have had to date. There are reviews to undertake, summaries to write, and findings to reach. By the end of this year, you may not know where you are heading, but you will certainly understand where you are now. At these junctures in our lives, we grow up a little bit more. And this is your year to become A Grown-Up Person. You are never too old to learn new tricks or make amends. You have these things going for you . . .

▶ Ⅴ Ⓦ *Naïveté. There are times when you must put your confidence completely in the hands of another. Call upon the trust you knew only as a child. Show them your real smile . . . and speak in your real voice.*

◀ Ⓐ Ⓦ *Experience. Everything you've ever done up till now counts—even what you don't remember. Call your entire experience set into play. Apply the lessons of your past to the things that need doing today.*

Ⓜ Ⓜ *Muscle. For the most part, you can depend on your body to get you to the places you need to go, even if it means lugging all your furniture with you. Don't just look at it, use your bulk.*

Ⓜ Ⓦ *Bone. Beneath the muscles, you are as brittle as an old bundle of bones. But no one needs to know your weakness, as long as you don't let it show. Most will never look more than skin deep, anyhow.*

Ⓗ Ⓗ ⮞ Ⓛ

9. Hail   21. Love

If you are 9, 21, 34, 46, 59, 71, 84, 96, or (Land o' Goshen!) 109, you have proved you can find your Runes. But can you clear the upcoming hurdles? You have come to a point in your life when both your wings and legs are tested. Will you hold up? Or be found lacking? This is a pivotal year. And I wouldn't be a bit surprised if it found you participating in some ancient rite of passage, for you are becoming a Whole Person. At any rate, you have a bridge to cross, and below it lies your Rubicon, Napoleon. In this ordeal there is no turning back once you have gotten your boots wet. No matter what your age in years, there are new stepping-stones to cross. At any rate, this year will teach you something you didn't already know—at least not about yourself. You have these things going for you . . .

Ⓗ Ⓗ *Tenacity. You have toes that hook, legs that lock, fingers that clutch, and arms that wrap. But it is your determination that makes you hang on for dear life. If you're falling, you can reach out and catch yourself.*

ᚱ ⏾ *Vitality. Draw your inspiration from the deep well within you. Replenish yourself. Renew your strength. Revive your spirit. You have the keys to the Fountain of Youth. Drink of the magic elixir.*

ᚴ ⊙ *Dreams. There is no one who worries more about you than your own subconsciousness. And there is no voice you have learned better to ignore. Take note of what your dreams say. Think about what the message could possibly be.*

ᚦ Ⓝ   **ᚷ Ⓧ**

10. Need   **22. beING**

If you are 10, 22, 35, 47, 60, 72, 85, 97, or (boy, oh boy!) 110, you have found your Runes. And I hope you're ready for them. It seems you've come to a point in your life when you need to explore your sexuality (again). As you may already know, it's also a good time for finding a new creative outlet, hobby, or other distracting interest. And if all else fails, I've heard cold showers work. What exactly happens during this frenzied year is more or less up to you. It all depends on your general orientation, personal preferences, tastes, moods, and, of course, the laws of your state. You are in the process of becoming a Contributing Human Being. Some will paint. Some will write. Some will make beautiful music together. Some will sing a cappella. This year there is a good chance you will learn how to give freely. You will certainly learn how to express yourself. The first step is to acknowledge that you have needs. You have these things going for you . . .

ᚦ Ⓝ *Necessity. It's not really as if you have a choice about the feelings that you're feeling, or the urges that are egging you on, or the cravings that you crave. You can always say no, of course—but a hunger does not leave just because it's been denied. Nor is an itch satisfied for very long. You'll have to draw the line somewhere, I suppose. But it's certainly your own call.*

ᚷ Ⓧ *Invention. You can read the Kamasutra to your heart's content, but all you'll ever learn are the names of parts and how to do things by the numbers. Sex is an intimate experience that doesn't need a handbook* *or a lot of laws governing it. It's one of those things wherein . . . you can learn as you go.*

❙ ⓪   **✖ ⓪**

11. Ice   **23.** hOme

If you are 11, 23, 36, 48, 61, 73, 86, 98, or (good for you!) 111, you have found your section of the text. In fact, welcome home! You have come to a point in your life when you are ready to lock in, settle down, and snuggle in for the time being. You have stepped into your safety zones, dug your trenches, and erected your fences. You have strung out your property lines and hung your safety nets. And within this safe compound you have built, I see you cuddling up in your security blankets. You are in the process of becoming a Secure Person. But is this shelter of yours made of straw, sticks, or brick? And can it hold its own in a big wind? You'll have to wait and see. But for now, you might as well put the kettle on and bake a few gingerbread men. You have these things going for you . . .

❙ ⓪ *Propriety. To get along, you will have to measure up to "community standards," but not necessarily all of them . . . and certainly not all of the time. Usually it's a small price to pay. They say, without some rules there would be anarchy. But at the other extreme is dictatorship. You can still have your pick—but you better act quick.*

✖ ⓪ *Property. To get along with your neighbors, you may have to abstain from painting the outside purple or adding an hexagonal window to the garage. But you never have to come out except to get the mail, and you never have to invite them in.*

❖ ⓪ *Privacy. If people want to make videotapes of you through your windows, I guess that's their problem. Lucky you've got curtains. And just in case, I'd close them before getting entirely naked.*

◈ Ⓨ Ⓙ   **▷◁ ⓪**

12. Year   **24.** Destiny

If you are 12, 24, 37, 49, 62, 74, 87, 99, or (yes, indeed!) 112, you have looked up your age correctly. And you have come to a point in your life when things balance out. It's a time to wrap up loose ends, clean up shop, close the books, and unwind a little bit. This year will find you reaping the benefits of the things you started in the past. But even as you reap the rewards of your successes—or pay the price for your errors—you'll be making new resolutions (and vowing to keep them this time). You are in the process of becoming a Balanced Person. Good luck in all your endeavors. Keep the faith. Godspeed. You have these things going for you . . .

◇ ⟨Ø⟩ ⟨Ʌ⟩ ⟨J⟩ ⟨ſ⟩ *The Calendar. There are as many days as things to fit into them . . . and all the months of the year to keep you busy. You've got nothing but time on your hands. Yet every moment counts, especially the times you take off.*

▷◁ ⟨Ɖ⟩ ⟨Ɣ⟩ *The Clock. You have all the hours of the day and night to apportion to the tasks that you need to get out of the way. Use the hours as if they were dollars. And feel free to blow a couple every now and again.*

☐

25. weird

If you are 25, 50, 75, 100, or (jeepers-creepers!) 125, this is your answer. But it's weird. You've come to the point where everything old is new again. These are times when, despite your best efforts to keep things stable, they change. The unexpected has a way of happening this year. And you have no choice, except to make the most of it. The Universe pushes you around to where it wants you. And there is no stopping the world to get off. The developments that shape your life this year will set you on a whole new course and a brand-new adventure. You are in the process of becoming a Self-Made Person. Sometimes things have to get shaken up in order for us to get shaken loose. This, my friend, is one of those years. You have this going for you . . .

☐ *Nothing & Everything. All the doors are wide open. All the possibilities are in the hat. Nothing that hasn't happened yet is entirely certain. You have yet to write the next chapter.*

EXTRA CREDIT

How's it going? To find out, just mix up your Runes and think of your question: **What do I have going for me?** at work? in love? in life? Or think of your topic and say, **Tell me the skinny.** It also works if you simply say: **Speak!** Reach into your Runes and draw the three that feel wanted. Or cast a handful of Runes and pick three. Note whether each Rune is upside down or not. Then look it up in this Reading's Answer section, and read the *italic* text.

EXTRA, EXTRA CREDIT!

How to make a good-luck charm. For a special token of affection (or a great stocking stuffer), make your friends a lucky charm, marked with one of these traditional Runic symbols:

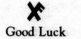
Good Luck

Eternal Love

Safe Home

You can make your token out of just about anything you have lying around. If you can woodwork: carve, sand, and stain. If you can sew: fold, stitch, or quilt. And if you can draw or paint, then seal or laminate.

Go on to the next Reading whenever you are ready to continue.

Reading #13

WHAT'S TO BECOME OF ME?
(Turn back the clock)

What does the old year have to teach? What does the new year hold in store? In this Reading, you will be using your Runes to get a rundown. The key is in your birth date. By drawing or casting Runes, you can also use this Reading to learn how to act now to undo a past mistake.

♪ ♪ ♪ ♪

RUNE TOOLS

Here's a summary chart of the Runes and their numbers. . . .

1	ᚠ F	7	ᚷ G	13	ᛖ Ē	19	ᛗ E
2	ᚢ U	8	ᚹ V W	14	ᛈ P	20	ᛗ M
3	ᚦ Th	9	ᚺ H	15	ᛉ Z	21	ᛚ L
4	ᚨ A	10	ᚾ N	16	ᛋ S	22	ᛝ X
5	ᚱ R	11	ᛁ I	17	ᛏ T	23	ᛟ O
6	ᚲ C K Q	12	ᛃ Y J	18	ᛒ B	24	ᛞ D

25 ᛩ

In Reading #12 we saw how the first twelve Runes can be paired with the second twelve. Rune pairs can also be formed by working frontwards and backwards through the Runic alphabet—pairing the first Rune with the 24th Rune, the second Rune with the 23rd, and so on. There are twelve of these pairs in all (reading top to bottom), ᚠ and ᛞ, ᚢ and ᛟ, ᚦ and ᛜ . . .

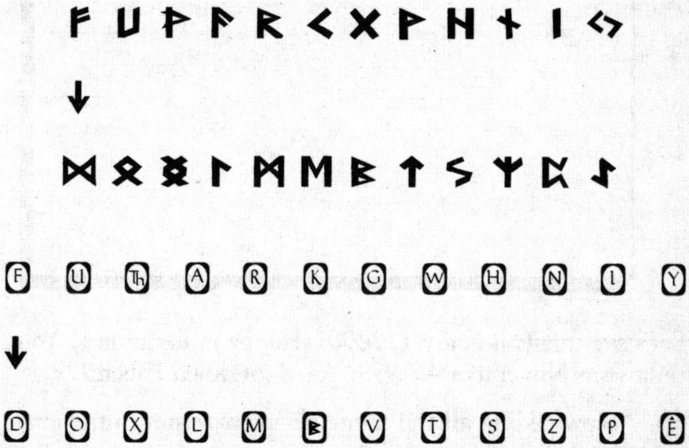
F U Th A R K G W H N I Y
D O X L M B V T S Z P Ê

The pairs formed in this way match up beautifully with one another, giving us a new way to read the Runes. In this Reading's Answer section, we'll be using these Rune pairs to chart your annual progress.

HOW TO

To get your forecast for the year ahead . . .

1 Just jot down the month, day, and year of your last birthday. (If you have a birthday coming up within six months, also jot it down.)

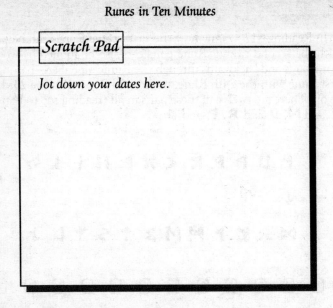

Scratch Pad

Jot down your dates here.

Let's say this is January 1, 2000. (Happy millennium!) Your last birthday was November 4, 1999. You'd jot down 11/4/1999.

2 Now add up all the numerals in this date. In the example: $1 + 1 + 4 + 1 + 9 + 9 + 9 = 34$.

3 If any date adds up to a number between 1 and 25, just look up your number in this Reading's Answer section.

If your number is larger than 25, subtract 25 from it, and look up the resulting number in the Answers. In the example, $34 - 25 = 9$. If the result is still higher than 25 at this point, subtract another 25. And keep subtracting by 25's until you have a number between 1 and 25. Then look up your Rune by its number.

You can also use this Reading for any other year, going as far back—or as far forward—as you like. You might want to try it with significant anniversaries, like the day you met, were married, or started a new job.

THE ANSWERS

The answers appear in the traditional order of the Runes, but they are listed in pairs. Reversed Runes immediately follow their upright counterparts (✕, ᚺ, ✝, ❘, ⟨⟩, ↑, ᛋ, ✿, ᛗ, and ☐ have no reversals).

F	U	Th	A	R	K	G	W	H	N	I	Y		
D	O	X	L	M	E	B	T	S	Z	P	Ê		O

ᚠ ᚢ ᚦ ᚨ ᚱ ᚲ ᚷ ᚹ ᚺ ᚾ ᛁ ⟨⟩
ᛗ ᛟ ᛨ ᛚ ᛗ ᛖ ᛒ ᛏ ᛋ ᛃ ᛈ ☐

K=C & Q; W=V; Y=J

ᚠ Ⓕ   ᛗ Ⓓ

1. Fortune   **24.** Destiny

The Year of the Blue Moon. This year is not necessarily a "once-in-a-lifetime" chance, but when it cycles up, my friend, it may feel like a rare opportunity. You are destined to succeed this year, particularly when it comes to money matters. If it is property you want, property you shall get. But power, status, and fame are also noble ambitions this year. Only health and love are outside your direct control right now. But if you find them too, you shall truly have it all before twelve moons have come and gone. Financial dealings are favored above all else. It's a time when you could even build a tidy nest egg. But at the very least, you won't end up in the hole. Here are the lessons you will walk away with . . .

ᚠ Ⓕ *You need to make money in order to spend it. But easy come, easy go, as they say. Let bygones be bygones.*

ᛞ Ⓓ *You need to invest money in order to make it grow. A penny saved is nothing earned. But who knows, in another 30 years . . .*

ᛗ Ⓓ Ⓓ *Your income needs to match your outflow in the end. Strike a balance between assets and liabilities. Compute net present value.*

ᚢ Ⓤ   ✿ Ⓞ

2. lUck   **23.** hOme

The Year of the Threshold. Whenever this year comes around, the emphasis will be on your residence or place of work. It's a good time for fixing up the old homestead, building a house of your own, setting up a bachelor pad, opening up a love nest, or even carrying your love across the threshold of a new life. It's also a good time to change jobs. It's a year for doing the groundwork and laying the cornerstone for your future security. Constructive projects of all kinds are encouraged. In one way or the other, you repitch your tent. Here are the lessons you could learn now . . .

ᚢ Ⓤ   *Count your blessings. Some do not even have a roof over their heads, let alone anything to come home to or anyone to meet them at the door.*

ᚾ Ⓝ   *Take the bad with the good . . . as long as the bad is not really all that bad . . . and as long as the good outweighs it.*

ᛉ Ⓞ   *Build your home on something firm, and be yourself constant and abiding to those who dwell with you.*

ᛉ Ⓞ   *A house turned upside down will be destroyed. But a home endures all attempts at destruction.*

ᚦ Ⓣⓗ   ᛉ Ⓧ

3. faiTh   **22. beING**

The Year of Thorns. Whenever this year rolls around, you can expect to get hung up on someone (or something) . . . stuck, snared, smitten—maybe even bitten! The year favors marriage, married life, and connubial relations of all kinds (provided, of course, that everyone involved is above the age of consent—and does). Heck, you might even tie the knot this year, renew your vows, or take new ones. Ironically enough, the year also favors celibates, virgins, and ascetics, who will get the chance to prove they can withstand the temptations of the flesh. It ought to be quite a year. Here are the lessons you could walk away with . . .

ᚦ Ⓣⓗ   *It's only natural to feel thorny. And you can deny it all you like—or indulge to your heart's content—but it just keeps coming back.*

◀ 🔲 *There is no such thing as uncomplicated sex. If it smells like a rose, it probably has thorns. (And if I were you, I wouldn't run naked through the woods.)*

✖ ⊠ *It usually takes two to tango . . . but someone's got to lead. (I believe it's your move.)*

⊩ Ⓐ　　　🔲 Ⓛ

4. fAte　　　21. Love

The Year of the Wellspring. When this year cycles back around, your heartstrings will have their periodic tug. And you will reach out for all kinds of love. But friendship, companionship, and camaraderie matter most to you now. So it's also a good time to renew old business acquaintances, get in touch with long-lost pals, or spend more time with the kids. The year favors going places, doing things, or just hanging out with one another. It's all very spontaneous . . . and in many respects, pleasantly ordinary. But looking back, this will be one of your all-time banner years. Here are the lessons you might learn . . .

⊩ Ⓐ *Fate brings you together. But the chemistry between you does the rest. The magic is either there or it's not.*

◢ Ⓥ *Fate takes you apart. But it was good while it lasted. And you can try to keep in touch.*

🔲 Ⓛ *Love's best words are spoken in a whisper. Love's best sound is a sigh. Love falls into place like an arrow that has hit its mark.*

◢ Ⓛ *Love takes back the words it said in anger at something else. Love forgives the hurt that was caused. But alas, love also has its falling out.*

🔲 Ⓡ　　🔲 Ⓜ

5. Reality　　　20. Male

The Year at the Crossroads. When this year cycles back around, you come to another juncture, junction, or turning point in your life. The road forks. Or suddenly you find yourself on what appears to be a detour. You get a gentle shove in a slightly different direction. A new avenue opens up. It's a year for reassessing your general direction, reviewing your accounts, and sizing things up. Not even long-standing relationships escape the inspection. Whatever it is you're looking for, it has something to do with "male reality." Perhaps you need to discover yours. Here's what you can expect to live and learn . . .

R Ⓡ *A man's car is an extension of his . . . self-image. But more telling is how fast he drives it . . . and how much he gets per gallon.*

↘ Ⓨ *Your wheels can take you places you've never been before . . . as long as you don't let the weather (or the radar) stop you.*

M Ⓜ *A man's gotta prove what a man's gotta prove . . . again and again and again, it seems . . . himself to himself. Meet your inner challenge.*

M Ⓦ *A real man knows how to be on the bottom, as well as on the top . . . how to fall with honor and how to get back up again with pride.*

‹ Ⓒ Ⓚ Ⓠ   **M** Ⓔ

6. Course,   **19. fEmale**
   Quest,
   Karma

The Year of the Fireworks. When this year cycles back around, you'll experience a sudden energy burst. There'll be plenty of hustle, lots of bustling around, and an incredible amount of hype going on. Events will trail by you so quickly, the sequence may become a blur. Yet from this chaos comes certainty. In random flashes—and with periodic booms—there'll be streaks of genius. It has something to do with a woman's ways of reaching conclusion. Perhaps you need to give expression to the woman within you—be you woman or man. Here's what you stand to learn once the dust is settled . . .

◀ ⊙ ⊙ ⊙ *To see things from a distance sometimes requires a telescope. But you'll still need to distinguish the mountain from the molehill.*

▶ ⊙ ⊙ ⊙ *To bring things into focus sometimes takes a magnifying glass. But you'll have to move the lens to see what's happening on the periphery.*

M ⊟ *A wise woman knows without knowing, sees without seeing, and tells without telling. Learn to listen as well as read.*

W ⊟ *A well-rounded woman knows how to put her pants on . . . one leg at a time. And in this case, one size fits all.*

✘ ⊙   ▶ ⊕

7. Gifts   **18.** Birth

The Year of the Child. When this year cycles up again, you'll feel rejuvenated . . . young again, new again, alive again, ready to begin again. It's a time for coming out of your shell, shedding your snakeskin (if you will), or emerging from your cocoon. New things are coming into being now. And one of them is you. Boy becomes man. Girl becomes woman. One takes the role of husband and father. One plays the part of wife and mother. And nobody can escape without having to change a diaper or two. It's a period of metamorphosis. You emerge as the new you. Here's what you stand the chance to learn . . .

✘ ⊙ ⊙ *Life is a surprise package. You never know what might be hidden deep down in the layers of tissue paper.*

▶ ⊕ *Birth is a process. Monitor the signs. Time the contractions with a stopwatch. Track the stages.*

◀ ⊙ *To be reborn is to be given another chance. It is better to build on the past than to discard it.*

ᚠ Ⓥ Ⓦ   ↑ Ⓣ

8. Wonder   **17. Triumph**

The Year of the Dragon. When this year cycles back around, you'll find yourself confronting your bugaboos. There are shadows to box with, illusions to jest with, and figments of the imagination to deal with. But not to fear! Tilting at windmills serves its purpose. And throwing a few false punches never hurt anyone. It's a time when triumph can come as if by magic. You might even find yourself thrust into the winner's circle. But at the very least you will feel a surge of glory, perhaps because you have confronted and overcome your own monsters. Here's what you might learn . . .

ᚠ Ⓥ Ⓦ *A victory of the self proving itself to itself is the sweetest, most glorious triumph known to man or woman . . . even if only you know what you have done.*

◀ Ⓐ Ⓦ *For everyone who wins, there is someone who loses. But would you rather be the champion or the contender?*

↑ Ⓣ *It's easier to fight a battle with weapons than it is with tools. But all's fair on the front lines . . . even psychological games.*

↓ Ⓘ *To be a trooper may require you to get your fatigues a little dirty. But all things considered, crawling on your belly is sometimes better than standing erect.*

ᚺ Ⓗ   ᛋ Ⓢ

9. Hail   **16. Sun & Stars**

The Year of the Hailstone. When this year cycles up, you need to be prepared for just about anything. The signs themselves are mixed. But it looks like there will be as many partly sunny days as mostly cloudy nights. You have no choice but to watch the storms roll in and pass away again, even if it means you have to modify your plans from day to day or run a little late. Everything cycles. And so do you. Now's your chance to get in sync with nature. At the very least, you will marvel at how these things all work out in their rightfully mysterious ways. Here's what you need to walk away with . . .

178

ᚺ Ⓗ *Though there are snow clouds in the sky and a nor'easter is blowing up the coast, know that the world is not ending. It is only weeding out.*

ᛋ Ⓢ *Watch for the Dog Star to return in summer and for Orion in the fall. The signs are there for you to read. See them. Study them. Know them.*

ᛏ Ⓝ   ᛉ Ⓩ

10. Need   **15. reSIStance**

The Year of the Locust. When this year cycles up again, you can look for some sweeping changes and more than a few major challenges. Some say that when you have your health, you've got it all. But this is a year when you will need your faith as much as or more than pills. There is much now to withstand, endure, and come through. And for the most part, you must bear this cross alone. But take heart. Though this is a difficult year, it is also a passable one. And in the end, it passes for a learning experience. What a difference a year can make, especially this one, especially to you. Here's what you can take from it . . .

ᛏ Ⓝ *Though hunger growls in your stomach and pain gnaws at your side, do not curse the day nor rue the night. Need wants much before it is satisfied. Consider it your sacrifice.*

ᛉ Ⓩ *If you would protect yourself from physical threat, there are ways to pump up both your strength and your courage. And neither comes from a bottle.*

ᛉ Ⓩ *If you would protect yourself from psychological damage, there are more ways than one to adjust your own attitude. If you feel like you're coming loose, tighten a few screws.*

ᛁ Ⓘ   ᛈ Ⓟ

11. Ice   **14. hoPe**

The Year of the Great White Hope. When this year cycles up, you will breathe a sigh of relief. Things may still look a little bleak right now, but conditions in general are starting to soften. And what held you in place will, on its own accord, set you free. There is something like a pregnant pause about this time. Things are still moving slowly. But the days of dragging are nearly over. All of a sudden, it will soon be as if it's always been 90 degrees in the shade and a cool 75 in the pool. While you wait for spring to follow winter, get ready to make your moves. Take these thoughts with you . . .

❘ ⓘ *Even when things slow to a standstill, there is reason to be confident, and there is progress to be made. If snow falls, ski. If ice forms, skate.*

◖ ⓟ *What would you have the future be? As your hand gropes among the Runes, you will know at least your wish. Now, how badly do you want it?*

◣ ⓓ *To see the future, you must accept the possibility of loss as well as gain. Life itself is a calculated risk. And you take your Runes in your own hand.*

◇ ⓨ ⓙ   **ↄ ⓔ**

12. Year   **13.** hElp

The Year of Years. When the twelfth year cycles up again, you come safely to the point of reconciliation. It is a year for giving thanks as well as making penance and atonement. You will be able to repay what you have borrowed. You will be able to make up for what you have done wrong. And you may even be able to earn yourself a few karmic brownie points in the process. This year will be an especially productive cycle for settling accounts. In some cases, a whole series of years will come to their natural conclusion over these next twelve months. The time teaches you this . . .

◇ ⓨ ⋀ ⓙ ⓕ *No matter how long the things you wait for take, the waiting finally passes, and the moment finally comes. Now, if only you could slow the hands of time!*

➽ 🄴 🄴 *It is only at the point of completion that one can know what it was all about. Now you can see what all your worry got you.*

🄾

25. weird

Year of the Big Leap. When this year cycles back around, it's kind of **weird**. But ain't we all? And ain't it grand? I figure the Universe must love diversity more than anything else, or why would we ever be living in a world like this? From the highest peaks to the ocean depths, it is nothing but a constant variation on an ever-popular theme. Be who you are, my friend. It's the only way you fit in. This is a year for taking a good long look in your magic mirror. And by now you ought to know what I mean. For it's not the body you want to admire—it's the eyes you need to look into. Next year a whole new cycle begins. Prepare yourself to make the big leap. Here's what you need to learn . . .

🄾 *Absolutely nothing is required of you now. Just wipe the slate clean, empty the ashtrays, and put out the trash.*

EXTRA CREDIT

To turn back the clock. If you'd like to know what you should have learned from some past experience—or what you can do to make up for it now—mix up your Runes while you ask: **What can I learn from _____?** Reach into your bag and draw the three Runes that work their way into your fingers. Or cast a handful of Runes on the ground and pick the three that your hand is attracted to. Note whether they are upright or reversed. Then look them up in this Reading's Answer section and consult the *italic* text. This method also works with questions about current or upcoming situations.

EXTRA, EXTRA CREDIT!

To make Decision Runes. Here's a dynamic way to zero in on a conclusion, using a special set of ancient Runes from the British Isles.

This method uses the same technique used by children to decide a point by playing the game Paper, Scissors, and Stone.

First, you'll need to make some special Runes out of sticks, stones, notepaper, buttons, or—what the heck—you can even use synthetic ivory. You'll need six lots in all. Write one of these Celtic symbols on one side of each of your lots (leaving one blank) . . .

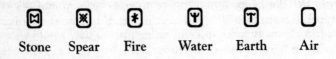

| Stone | Spear | Fire | Water | Earth | Air |

Or if you prefer, you can substitute your regular Runes for this activity . . .

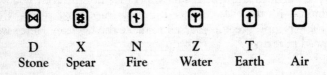

| D | X | N | Z | T | |
| Stone | Spear | Fire | Water | Earth | Air |

While you mix up your Decision Stones, think about the issue you are trying to resolve. Now select two stones. The object is to think about the relationship that exists between the two symbols and draw your own conclusions, but here are some suggested interpretations . . .

Stone deflects Spear, resists Fire, sheds Water, returns to Earth, falls through Air.

Spear is sharpened by Stone, reinforced by Fire, rusted by Water, cleansed by Earth, and unresisted by Air.

Fire cracks Stone, softens Spear, heats Water, bakes Earth, and smokes up the Air.

Water smooths Stone, slows Spear, extinguishes Fire, runs off Earth, and evaporates into Air.

T   Earth conceals Stone, accepts Spear, puts out Fire, turns Water to mud, and dusts up the Air.

O   Air shapes Stone, carries Spear, encourages Fire, stirs Water, and kicks up Earth.

Go on to the next Reading whenever you are ready to continue.

Reading #14

WHO IS MY COMPANION?
(Tell the truth about us)

Is he right for you? Will she stand by you through and through?
Where's this whole thing headed, anyway? In this Reading you'll
draw or cast your Runes to see if the two of you are meant to be
. . . and if it's forever.

ᛉ ᛉ ᛉ

RUNE TOOLS

Every Rune has a "double" . . . a Rune that serves as its companion
in the set. You've already worked with these doubles in Reading #11,
where we matched them up with the Zodiac signs. As you can see
from the chart, each Rune also has a "gender," male ♂ or female ♀.

THE RUNES AND THEIR GENDER

Pairs	♂	♀	♂	♀	
1.	ᚠ	ᚢ	Ⓕ	Ⓤ	
2.	ᚦ	ᚨ	Ⓣⓗ	Ⓐ	
3.	ᚱ	ᚲ	Ⓡ	Ⓒ Ⓚ	Ⓠ
4.	ᚷ	ᚹ	Ⓖ	Ⓥ	Ⓦ
5.	ᚺ	ᚾ	Ⓗ	Ⓝ	
6.	ᛁ	ᛃ	Ⓘ	Ⓨ	Ⓙ

Pairs	♂	♀	♂	♀
7.	↑	⋈	Ê	P
8.	↑	⟨	Z	S
9.	↑	B	T	B
10.	M	⋈	E	M
11.	↑	⋈	L	X
12.	⋈	⋈	O	D
	☐	☐	☐	☐

We'll be using these male and female Runes to help you seek your mate, a lover, companion, or friend . . . or reconfirm you've found the right one.

HOW TO

To find out whether a relationship is right for you . . .

1 Separate your Runes into two piles of twelve Runes each. Make one pile of "male" Runes (ᚠᚦᚱᚷᚺᛁᛃᛇᛏᛗᛚᛜ). Make another pile of "female" Runes (ᚢᚠᚲᛈᛏᛟᚾᛊᛒ ᛖᛜᛞ). Place the Blank Rune in the pile of your choice. (If you line up all your Runes in Futhark order first, separating them into the two piles will be a snap.) To use alphabet tiles instead, consult the chart in the Tools section to identify the English letters that are male and female.

2 Mix up each pile of Runes (or letters) separately. Close your eyes if you like. Think of the person in your life. Ask: **Is it meant to be for us?** Select one Rune from the appropriate pile of male or female Runes—first for you and then for the other person.[1] This Reading also works with questions like: **How do things stand**

---

[1] For gay and lesbian readers: Just choose both Runes from the same pile.

between us? in general? at this moment? **How will this relationship wind up?** Or simply: **Are we right for each other?** You can also try it with platonic relationships or close friendships (but be prepared to laugh).

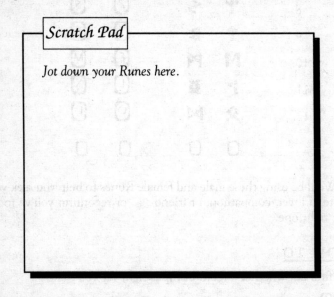

Scratch Pad

Jot down your Runes here.

3 Note whether each Rune is upside down or right side up. Then look up both Runes in this Reading's Answer section. For the first Rune you selected, read the YOU section of the text. For the second Rune you selected, read the HIM or HER section of the text. Or, for a more complete answer, you can read the whole text for each Rune.

THE ANSWERS

The answers appear in the traditional order of the Runes. Reversed Runes immediately follow their upright counterparts (✗, ᚺ, ✚, ᛁ, ◇, ↑, ⌉, ✸, ᛗ, and ▯ have no reversals).

F U Th A R K G W H N I Y Ê P Z S T B E M L X O D

ᚠ ᚢ ᚦ ᚠ ᚱ ᚲ ᚷ ᚹ ᚺ ✚ ᛁ ◇ ᛃ ⟨⟩ ᚲ � ᛋ ↑ ᛒ ᛖ ᛗ ᛘ ᛚ ᚷ ᛟ ᛞ

▯ The Blank Rune appears last.   K=C & Q; W=V; Y=J

ᚠ Ⓕ

Fortune

YOU—Since you are a man of fortune, you may not have the time for a full-blown relationship. The look of the woman on your arm may be more important to you than who she is. You are more in the market for a car than a wife.

HIM—He is a man of fortune. So a marriage of convenience would suit him fine. All the better if you bring along a nice dowry of your own. Prospects are good you will live well—even if it's mostly on your money.

ᛄ Ⓕ

Fortune reversed

YOU—Because you are a man of few means, you can't give her everything she wants, needs, or deserves. But as long as you stick together and believe in each other, you will have far more than worldly goods.

HIM—He is a man of misfortune. So there is nothing but love and romance to be gained from marrying him. But one could do worse than be poor and happy.

ᚢ Ⓤ

lUck

YOU—Since you're lucky at love in general, you may not fully appreciate what you've got here. Even if it seems too good to be true, you can never be sure until you give it a fair chance. You're looking for Mr. Right.

HER—She feels like the luckiest woman alive—and it's all because of you. Just keep doing what you're doing. But if you want to keep her, you will have to be true.

ᚾ ⓝ

lUck reversed

YOU—You think you're pretty lucky to have caught this one. And I think you're right. Luck—even when it's reversed—has a way of being all right. I'd say the odds are in your favor.

HER—She's happy-go-lucky . . . but only when it comes to you. So don't get the wrong idea. Look, pal, you've gotten more than lucky this time. So don't blow it.

ᚦ ⓣⓗ

faiTh

YOU—You're looking for someone who's interested in you and only you. For you demand fidelity above all else. You want someone who is devoted exclusively to you. You are looking for a permanent relationship.

HIM—He simply adores you and would do anything for you. You may even have him eating out of your hand before soon! When on bended knee he comes to pop the question, what will your answer be?

ᚦ ⓣⓗ

faiTh reversed

YOU—You've been a busy boy, haven't you? Okay, so it wasn't exactly being "unfaithful," but you'd never convince a jury, now would you? Call it all off while you still can. And quit thinking with your you-know-what.

HIM—Well, he has eyes, all right . . . but they're not exactly glued to one spot, if you know what I mean. Well, let him look. If we weren't all tempted, fidelity wouldn't be such great shakes.

ᚠ Ⓐ

fAte

YOU—You feel as if this is one of those things that was simply meant to be. The gods have spoken, as it were. Kind of funny, isn't it—when you were looking for something entirely different.

HER—She feels fatalistic about you, which is either good or bad. You are either the man of her dreams or the focus of her worries. (More than likely, it's a little of the two.)

ᚠ Ⓥ

fAte reversed

YOU—You feel as if something has caught up to you. Perhaps it is something from the past that haunts you—or is it some<u>one</u>? It is time to make amends, put this behind you, and move on.

HER—She feels that if it wasn't meant to be, it just wasn't. If you feel the same way, so be it. But if not, you might still have a chance. Go to her now with your tail between your legs and flowers behind your back. Woo her.

ᚱ Ⓡ

Reality

YOU—As a realist, you already see this relationship for what is. If not, you must be careful to observe. It is not only what meets the eye, you know. You are looking for something more than skin-deep.

HIM—He's quiet sometimes, and difficult to read. But then suddenly he will turn and blurt out the truth. He's a realist, you know, and it sometimes hurts. But in the end he makes up for it.

ᚱ Ⓨ

Reality reversed

YOU—As a surrealist, you can't always see things in their proper perspective. This relationship has your senses bent out of shape, as it were. And you feel more or less head over heels.

HIM—He's mad about you . . . and I mean that in the nicest way. He can't get you out of his mind. He can't quit thinking of you. You have him bothered to the point of distraction. Be kind to him.

< ⟨ ⟩ ⟨ ⟩ ⟨ ⟩

Course, Quest, Karma

YOU—You already know the answer to this one. Your feelings about the relationship are simply right. Whatever happens, rest assured it's destined. You are looking for your soul mate.

HER—She feels about you the same way you feel about her. It's either the real thing or it's not. And in this case, you have to go with your intuition. I think you know what I'm talking about.

> ⟨ ⟩ ⟨ ⟩ ⟨ ⟩

Course, Quest, Karma reversed

YOU—You're totally in the dark about this one, aren't you? Well, sometimes you have to be hit over the head to see the light (just kidding). Let me say this: When you finally get the message, it's gonna melt your cheese.

HER—She can't figure you out. Ah, but that's the attraction! She likes the strong, silent type. Open your eyes, pal. What are you waiting for? Wake up and hear the cat meow.

✕ ⟨ ⟩ ⟨ ⟩

Gifts

YOU—You feel as if you have found your "significant other." And you want to give yourself to her . . . hopefully for a long time. You are looking to make a commitment.

HIM—He feels like he wants to sign his name at the X and commit himself to you. (Is that why he's bringing you all those presents?) At any rate, it is the thoughts that count—and his are fixed on you.

ᚠ ⓥ ⓦ

Wonder

YOU—You feel like you are about to burst wide open with the feelings you feel. Wow! What can I tell you that you don't already know? Is it the real thing? At this point, who cares? You're looking for what you've already found.

HER—She lights up your life. And when she passes through the room, you heart palpitates with joy . . . if you know what I mean. (Pal, is that a gun in your pocket?) Go on, ask her to dance.

ᚨ ⓐ ⓦ

Wonder reversed

YOU—You feel like you can't keep this feeling inside you anymore or you will simply burst. How could you hope to contain something of this magnitude? Come on, pal, let your feelings out.

HER—She'd like to hear the words that you have such difficulty saying. And you know the words I mean. Repeat after me: "I love you, honey muffin."

ᚺ ⓗ

Hail

YOU—You've been arguing, or something. Things look pretty dark and dangerous. Well, most relationships have a few sparks (or there would be no sparkle). Apologize whether you're right or wrong. Maybe it'll all blow over.

HIM—He's disturbed about something. Perhaps you had a little tiff—maybe even an all-out blowout. Maybe he's really upset about something else. Or maybe he just has a short fuse. Talk it over. Try working it out.

ᛏ ⓝ

Need

YOU—You feel this burning desire and an incredible urge to play with fire. But you also have many other needs that need to be met.

So it's good in bed. . . . How else is it? Sometimes you just want to be held.

HER—She's got the hots for you, all right. But are you sure you know what you're getting into? Are you sure you're willing to be there when she <u>really</u> needs you? Like now?

▌ ⏇

Ice

YOU—Looks to me like you're getting the cold treatment. So you must have done <u>something</u>. Or maybe you're just barking up the wrong tree. Either make up or take a hike. You're looking for something warm and nice.

HIM—He can be pretty dense sometimes—maybe even as thick as a brick—and hard to get to know. You'll have to get through to him somehow. When all else fails, light a fire under him.

◇ ⏃ ⏃ ⏃ ⏃

Year

YOU—You've had to work pretty hard at this relationship. And only you can say whether it was worth it or not. But what you have now is just about as good as it will ever get. You want to be in it for the long term.

HER—She's perfect for you. And she's waited long enough to hear the words from your lips. Tell her how you feel. Make her day, week, month, and year.

⏚ ⏃ ⏃

hElp

YOU—You're in this one, pal, for better or worse, richer or poorer, in sickness and in health. And with this Rune in your pocket, you will stay true to your word. You want something that lasts.

HIM—He's never even looked at another woman—well, at least not <u>really</u>. He wants you and only you. And if you give him half a chance, he'll prove he means it.

⚐ ⓟ

hoPe

YOU—You're willing to go all the way, roll those high dice, and win big. And don't you deny it. Hey, if I were you, I'd take the risk. What have you got to lose? It's worth a shot, isn't it?

HER—She's got your number. She knows where you live. And one of these days she's going to be coming to see you. So if I were you, I'd tidy up and change the sheets.

⚐ ⓓ

hoPe reversed

YOU—You wish! Well, it's worth a try. But you'll need to take the risk of being disappointed in the process. You never know, though. So go ahead—take your chances. It's up to you. Here's hoping you luck out this time.

HER—She's trouble—but that's part of the attraction, isn't it? And you never know which way she will go or what she might do next. How much of a gambler are you? These are pretty big stakes.

Ⲙ ⓩ

reSIStance

YOU—You're feeling pretty protective about this one. Someone either needs to be fought for or fended off. Either way, I'd say it's fairly serious. You're looking out for someone. You're fighting for something.

HIM—This guy knows how to take care of himself . . . and, by extension, you. It's nice to feel his strong arms around you. It's nice to have him around for protection. (Just be sure he wears some.)

⚔ ⓩ

reSIStance reversed

YOU—You're willing to let this one go . . . to throw down your sword (as it were) and call it a day. Well, so what? It was a knock-down, drag-out, wasn't it? And you need a break.

HIM—This guy is vulnerable right now, so give him the benefit of your doubt, but no more than that. You can't take in every sick puppy that comes along, you know. Some will run away as soon as they are well.

↘ Ⓢ

Sun & Stars

YOU—You have stars in your eyes over this one. But can life be all sunsets and moonlit walks? Of course not. But at least this relationship does have its moments. You're looking for a wishing star.

HER—She lights up your life . . . turns dark into day and makes you wish the nights could last forever. She takes your breath away. (Be still, my beating heart.)

↑ Ⓣ

Triumph

YOU—You'd like to conquer quickly and get out just as fast as you can zip up your pants. But when you have someone in every port, do you really have anyone? In fact, you are mostly interested in the chase.

HIM—You've found yourself a winner this time. But how will you ever compete with the big game? And when he comes home, how will you know where he's been?

↓ Ⓣ

Triumph reversed

YOU—You'd like to surrender completely . . . if you only could. And I'm not necessarily talking about throwing in the towel. You're looking for someone to take care of you and nurse you back to health.

HIM—He's given up . . . to you. So as the victor, I guess you can decide how to divide up the spoils. For this round—at least—you're the winner, so you get to do things your way. Show mercy.

ʁ ⑥

Birth

YOU—You would like to have children. And even though time may not be running out, you feel instinctively that it's time to get started. There are worse reasons for entering a relationship. You are looking for a family.

HER—She's pregnant! Or, at the very least, she would not be the least upset to be. So how do you feel about it? Are you ready for children? (Can anyone ever be?)

◄ ⑨

Birth reversed

YOU—You'd rather not have children . . . at least not right now. But there may be no choice for you, depending on the law and your own better judgment.

HER—She's not pregnant! Which may come as a relief to you . . . or a disappointment. There are many mouths to feed already in the world and many spirits to nourish. She'll be okay. And so will you.

M ⑥

fEmale

YOU—You feel a soft spot in your gut. You feel the gentle tugging at your heart. Lust or love—you should know the difference by now. So why would you doubt? You're not looking for just anyone, are you?

HIM—He's an open book—at least when it comes to telling you how he feels about you. So if you were looking for a courting, this sure should do the trick. If you let him, he will sweep you off your feet.

W ⑥

fEmale reversed

YOU—You don't know what you feel. And besides, you're not paying attention. You don't look into your head for the answers to questions like this one. The truth of this matter defies all rhyme and reason. It can only be intuited.

HIM—He's at a loss when it comes to expressing his feelings. So what are you going to do? With him it's all numbers and logic. If you want to reach him at all, you'll have to meet him halfway.

ᛗ Ⓜ

Male

YOU—You know your own mind. And this one measures up . . . at least to some of your criteria. The little things can always be changed. So why not? You're looking for something to build on.

HER—She has you just where she wants you. (Or is it the other way around?) At any rate, now that everyone's suited up and in position, let the games begin!

ᛗ Ⓦ

Male reversed

YOU—You know what you're feeling about this one. But how many times have your feelings deceived you before? It's pause for thought, I suppose. But every once in a while they are right on. This is one of those times.

HER—She relates to you . . . on some level that's difficult to describe. It's as if she knows you better than you know yourself. (And you better believe it, pal.)

ᛚ Ⓛ

Love

YOU—You are in love. Aye, me! And it's just like they say. You are like Romeo picking roses . . . throwing stones at Juliet's window . . . climbing up to her balcony. You also are like to pine away.

HIM—He's like a puppy dog. And if you would just blow in his ear, you'd have him rolled over on his back and windmilling his hind leg uncontrollably. Be gentle, my dear—he may prove ticklish.

◣ ⑦

Love reversed

YOU—You are in love. No. Yes. No. Yes. Oh . . . pal! She loves you. She loves you not. Who was it who said life's a rollercoaster? Well, they were wrong, it's love that makes you want to throw up your hands and scream.

HIM—He's vacillating . . . again. His feet are cold, perhaps? Well, I give it 24 to 36 hours and he should be back under your balcony again. I'd say this is more than puppy love. He'll come around.

✖ Ⓧ

beING

YOU—The two of you really ought to come up for air once in a while. I feel I should say that passionate hugs and kisses can only take you so far—but I'd hate to interrupt the mood.

HER—She wants to bleep your brains out, pal. So if you think you're man enough, the motel always has a vacancy. (But if I were you, I wouldn't pay for a room with a view.)

✖ Ⓞ

hOme

YOU—You want to move in together—but will it be your place or hers? What you really need is a little place where you can spend your days and nights together. You're looking to have it all.

HIM—He wants to live with you. And that's usually a good sign. All that's left to decide is whether you want to live with him. I'll leave it up to you.

✖ Ⓞ

hOme reversed

YOU—You want to pick up roots and move on. Well, every bird's gotta fly sometime. And I guess your time has come. Try to do it gracefully and be considerate of those who are behind and below you.

HIM—He wants to make a new home. Or else he wants to sell the house and buy a camper with a shower and a toilet that flushes blue. You'd better stay apprised of what he's thinking.

ᛗ ◻ ◻

Destiny

YOU—Your meeting was predestined. What's done is done. What's past is gone. This is how it is, was, and ever shall be. You're done looking . . . at least for this one.

HER—She was made for you. You are two proverbial peas in a pod. But what you've had so far has run its initial course. It's time to go on to the next step. What happens now is your joint decision.

◻

weird

YOU—This is **weird**. And I regret to report that this relationship was finished before its start. Perhaps you are looking too hard . . . or in the wrong heart.

THEM—They are out there by the droves . . . and one of them is waiting to catch your eye. Try to choose better and wiser this time. The decision is yours.

EXTRA CREDIT

To learn the truth about a relationship. Divide out your Runes as described in this Reading's How To section. As you think of the person you are—or were—involved with, say, **Tell the truth about us.** Draw two Runes from the pile of Runes for your gender. Then draw three more from the Runes for your partner's gender. In the order your drew them, place them in this classic formation, sometimes known as Thor's Cross:

```
        1
      2 5 4
        3
```

Look up each Rune in this Reading's Answer section. The first two Runes you selected describe you, so read the YOU portion of the answers. Runes 3 and 4 describe the other person, so read the HIM or HER description, as fits. Finally, for the 5th Rune, read both parts of the answer.

EXTRA, EXTRA CREDIT!

To make a significator Rune. When reading the Runes for others, some people like to put a Rune on the table to signify the person being read for. This significator Rune serves as the focal point for the reader, and has no separate meaning of its own. Though not necessary, it's kind of a magical touch that may also improve your concentration, and therefore your results.

To make a significator Rune, just find yourself one object that is similar to the other Runes in your set. (Add one matchstick, Popsicle stick, stone, or other gadget of your choice.) Use paint, pen, or marker and draw the symbol for "female" on one side, and the symbol for "male" on the other:

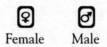

Female   Male

À la Kazam! You're ready to go to work. To use your new Rune, just turn it out first at the start of a Reading, male-side up if reading for a man and female side up when reading for a woman. Concentrate on it while you mix up your Runes in order to bring focus, sharpness, and clarity to the session. As you draw Runes for the layout, just arrange them around the significator, however you like . . .

♂

♀

[1] [2] [3]   [3] [2] [1]

A variation on this theme is to simply add two different objects to your Rune kit, say an oblong stone for the male and an oval stone for the female.[2]

Go on to the next Reading whenever you are ready to continue.

[2] Thanks to P. M. H. Atwater (*The Magical Language of Runes*, Bear & Company, 1986).

Reading #15

WHERE ARE MY FRIENDS?
(Double, double, take my trouble)

In this Reading, you'll draw or cast your Runes to find out who your true friends are . . . and are not. You can also use this Reading to think about where a particular friendship is headed in the long run. To get out of a jam, consult the Extra, Extra Credit section.

ᛉᛉᛉ

RUNE TOOLS

As we saw in Reading #12, the 24 Runes of the Elder Futhark can be divided into two halves of 12 Runes each. The first 12 can then be matched with the second 12 to form 12 pairs . . .

PAIRS	RUNES		TILES			
1.	ᚠ ᛊ		(F)			(Ē)
2.	ᚢ ᚴ		(U)			(P)
3.	ᚦ ᛉ		(Th)			(Z)
4.	ᚨ ᛋ		(A)			(S)
5.	ᚱ ᛏ		(R)			(T)
6.	ᚲ ᛒ		(C) (K)	(Q)		(B)
7.	ᚷ ᛗ		(G)			(E)

201

PAIRS	RUNES		TILES		
8.	ᚱ	ᛗ	Ⓥ Ⓦ		Ⓜ
9.	ᚺ	ᛁ	Ⓗ		Ⓛ
10.	ᛏ	ᛟ	Ⓝ		Ⓧ
11.	ᛁ	ᛉ	Ⓘ		Ⓞ
12.	ᛇ	ᛝ	Ⓨ Ⓙ		Ⓓ

In this Reading, when you draw one Rune, you'll actually be drawing two: the Rune itself and its equivalent Rune from the other half of the alphabet. Together they will give you your answers.

HOW TO

To find out who your friends are . . .

① Sort out your Runes into two piles. Into the first pile place the first 12 Runes in the Futhark sequence (ᚠᚢᚦᚨᚱᚲᚷ ᚹᚺᚾᛁᛇ). This will leave you with 12 Runes for the second pile (ᛈᛉᛊᛏᛒᛖᛗᛚᛜᛟᛞᛝ). Place the Blank Rune in the pile of your choice. To use alphabet tiles instead, just consult the table in the Tools section, and sort out your letters accordingly.

② Now mix up the Runes in the first pile while you think of the person you want to ask about. Ask your question: **Is so-and-so a friend of mine?** right now? will they be? or **What kind of a friend is _____?** Run your hands through your Runes and find the one that you will. Note whether it is upright or reversed. Repeat your question and draw a Rune from the second pile of Runes, placing it beside the Rune you drew before.

```
┌─────────────────┐
│  Scratch Pad    │
└─────────────────┘

Jot down your Runes here.
```

3   Look up both your Runes in this Reading's Answer section. For each Rune you have drawn, read the main text, then follow the *See Also* reference to the "equivalent" Rune and read its *italic* text. Together these two passages will give you the entire answer for each Rune.

THE ANSWERS

The answers appear in the traditional order of the Runes. Reversed Runes immediately follow their upright counterparts (✕, ᚺ, ✝, ᛁ, ‹›, ᛋ, ᛌ, ᛉ, ᛗ, and ☐ have no reversals).

F U Th A R K G W H N I Y Ê P Z S T B E M L X O D

ᚠ ᚢ ᚦ   ᚠ ᚱ ᚲ ᚷ   ᚹ ᚺ ✝ ᛁ ‹› ᛋ ᚲ ᛃ ↑ ᛒ ᛗ ᛗ ᛚ ᛦ ᚷ ᛞ

☐   The Blank Rune appears last.   K=C & Q; W=V; Y=J

ᚠ Ⓕ

Fortune

ON THE SURFACE—It would look like they are only in it for the money. So if their interest seems self-serving, it probably is. How would they behave toward you if there were nothing to gain? *See also* **ᚾ**—*hElp*.

At the start, you were taken in by appearances. But then you got to know each other. And in the final analysis, the lasting impressions were correct.

ᚠ Ⓕ

Fortune reversed

UNDERNEATH—Gain is the furthest thing from their mind. So if you think they've been after you for something, perhaps it's only a kiss and a hug. If you suspect ulterior motives, in this case there are none. *See also* **ᚾ**—*hElp*.

In the beginning, you had common goals and mutual interests. Along the way you encouraged each other greatly. By the end you each will have made it on your own.

ᚢ Ⓤ

lUck

ON THE SURFACE—They act as if they are lucky to know you. (And I agree.) So, unless you have some solid reason for doubting their intentions, I'd say you've lucked out this time. *See also* **ᚲ**—*hoPe*.

In the beginning, your paths crossed. Then you went along for the ride together. But in the end you are each responsible for your own deeds.

ᚿ Ⓤ

lUck reversed

UNDERNEATH—They think you are testing your luck. But is it any of their business? If so, listen patiently to their good advice. If not, do as you will—but never in spite. *See also* **ᚴ**—*hoPe reversed*.

At the start, it seemed to be in the cards. Then each of you played your separate hands. But in the end, only one can win.

⮞ 🜔

faiTh

ON THE SURFACE—They act as if they think you can walk on water. That's why they are constantly singing your praises. If you can't believe what they say to your face, then who can you trust? *See also* Ⓨ—*reSIStance.*

At the outset, you had the same ideas. But experience molded each of you. And by the end, you will have each expressed yourself differently.

◀ 🜔

faiTh reversed

UNDERNEATH—They have their doubts about you. Perhaps it was something you did to blemish your own image or tarnish your good name. You will have to prove yourself if you want to be back in their good graces again. *See also* ⮚—*reSIStance reversed.*

At the start, you believed everything you were told. But along the way you developed opinions of your own. By the end, you will have read between the lines enough to defend your position.

⮞ Ⓐ

fAte

ON THE SURFACE—They are glad your paths have crossed. And you can take them at their word for that, for their actions speak the same truth. You are part of each other's experience. *See also* ⮜—*Sun & Stars.*

From the start, it just happened. And as it unfolded, you went with the flow. But it was only later that you could appreciate it. By the end you will have accepted it for what it is.

↙ Ⓥ

fAte reversed

UNDERNEATH—They wonder why the two of you must be apart. And there is no good answer for this. The time has just come to move on. The time has come to go. Adieu. *See also* ⟩—*Sun & Stars.*

From the start, it was never meant to last forever. That's one of the things that made it taste so sweet. By the end, it leaves you with a tear on your cheek—but it is one worth shedding.

↖ Ⓡ

Reality

ON THE SURFACE—They see you for what you are . . . and appear to accept it. With them, too, what you see is what you get. You must ask yourself, who would you rather be with? *See also* ↑—*Triumph.*

From the start, you were both looking for something. For a while you did your "own thing" together. By the end, you will have each found your own version of the same truth.

↙ Ⓡ

Reality reversed

UNDERNEATH—They want you to be something you are not— and that's unfortunate. The two of you are like old dogs set in their respective ways. You have two different views of reality. Can the two ever possibly mesh? *See also* ↓—*Triumph reversed.*

From the start, you were headed in different directions. You shared the same dream for a time. And by the end, you will have each continued on your own separate ways.

◀ Ⓒ Ⓝ Ⓠ

Course, Quest, Karma

ON THE SURFACE—They depend on you to guide them, O enlightened one. So you must do your best to live up to their high expectations. To keep their respect, you must give them good advice. *See also* **ᛒ**—*Birth*.

From the start, the chemistry was right. You were their fearless leader for a while. But then—as you are inclined to do—you had a new idea. In the end, your influence will continue.

> ⟨⟩ ⟨⟩ ⟨⟩

Course, Quest, Karma reversed

UNDERNEATH—They would like to see you exposed for what you are. So if you have something to hide, you'd better hide it well and not get caught in the act. Someone's keeping tabs on you. *See also* **◀**—*Birth reversed*.

From the start, you did not like the looks of each other. And it was all downhill from there. But by the end, you will have each found your respective corner of the Universe.

✕ ⟨⟩ ⟨⟩

Gifts

ON THE SURFACE & UNDERNEATH—They are genuinely glad to know you. In their eyes, you are God's gift—and you can do no wrong. If you're really lucky, you feel the same way about them. *If you are a woman, see also* **M**—*fEmale. If you are a man, see* **W**—*fEmale reversed*.

From the start, you admired each other's gifts. In the interim you exchanged a few. And by the time it's all said and done, you will have come pretty close to breaking even.

ᚠ ⟨V⟩ ⟨W⟩

Wonder

ON THE SURFACE—They are happy to be in your company. So rest assured the hearty greeting you exchange is felt both ways. You can shake hands on it. You can even punch each other in the ribs. *See also* **M**—*Male*.

From the start, you hit it off. It continued in much the same way as it began. And by the end, you will have shared more than a few laughs together.

◀ ◊ ᛗ

Wonder reversed

UNDERNEATH—They are happy with you, but in a rather restrained way. So don't expect many public displays of affection. And don't be looking for praise. Still, they care deeply about you. See also **ᛉ**—*Male reversed*.

At the start, you were both unhappy. But then, at least you shared in that. And by the time it is all over, you will surely look back fondly on your bittersweet acquaintance.

ᚺ ⊞

Hail

ON THE SURFACE & UNDERNEATH—They are true to the end. And—believe you me—they will stand by you come hell or high water. When push comes to shove, they will be there—even in the darkest hours. See also **ᚱ**—*Love and* **◀**—*Love reversed*.

From the start, conditions have been variable. Every now and again all hell breaks loose. But there are long, silent lulls, as well. By the end, everything will have come out in the wash.

✚ ℕ

Need

ON THE SURFACE & UNDERNEATH—They need you . . . pure and simply, it's as easy as that. They are depending on you. So you need to show up and get the job done. Be there. See also **ᛝ**—*beING*.

From the start, it's been a mutually beneficial relationship. You scratched each other's backs along the way. And by the end, you will have helped each other make it through the shortest days . . . as well as the longest nights.

Ⅰ **Ⓘ**

Ice

ON THE SURFACE & UNDERNEATH—They feel loyal to you. But they're not exactly sure why. It could be a sense of dedication or a fearful respect, I suppose. At any rate, there is something very solid here, even if it sometimes feels rather cold. *See also* **✖**—*hOme and* **✖**—*hOme reversed.*

At the start, things were stiff and professional. But as you got to know each other better, the ice broke. By the end you will have melted together and melded into one heart.

⟨⟩ Ⓨ Ⓐ Ⓙ Ⓡ

Year

ON THE SURFACE & UNDERNEATH—They want it all to work out with you. But these things take time. And nothing was accomplished overnight—except a good night's sleep. Get yourself one, and carry on tomorrow. *See also* **⋈** —*Destiny.*

At the start, you both had the same objective. Your common goals brought you closer. And by the end, you will have done something more together than you ever imagined on your own.

↓ Ⓔ Ⓔ

hElp

UNDERNEATH & ON THE SURFACE—They want to help you. So if you need help, all well and good—take it. But if you don't, don't. Do think about it, though. And don't be unnecessarily proud. *See also* **ᚠ** —*Fortune and* **◢**—*Fortune reversed.*

From the beginning, one of you has needed protection. All along, you have lent each other a hand. And by the end, you will have done an even number of favors.

209

ᚸ Ⓟ

hoPe

UNDERNEATH—They are rooting for you all the way. So if you needed a cheering section, you've got one now. Here's hoping with them that you can beat the odds. *See also* ᚢ *—lUck.*

From the start, you've been taking your chances. And in the interim, you've scored as well as erred. But until it's all over, there is always a prayer. By the end, yours will be answered.

ᚴ Ⓓ

hoPe reversed

ON THE SURFACE—They are betting against you. But they have no way of knowing how the dice you are rolling will land. So don't let them psyche you out with their doomsday prophecies. Spin the wheel with confidence. *See also* ᚾ *—lUck reversed.*

From the start, the odds were against you. But it didn't stop you before and it shouldn't stop you now. By the end, it will be clear—at last—who was wrong and who was right.

ᛉ Ⓩ

reSIStance

UNDERNEATH—They want to protect you. Why else would they be making the sign of the cross over you? Take their blessings and well-wishes in the spirit intended. Let them feel as if they are taking care of you. *See also* ᚦ *—faiTh.*

From the start, you have looked out for each other. All along, you stuck together through thick and thin. And—by George—you will remain true to the bitter end.

ᛣ Ⓩ

reSIStance reversed

ON THE SURFACE—They regard you as a threat. Why else would they be burning a cross in your yard and chanting "work of

210

the devil"? The only thing to do is minimize your exposure to such negative influences. *See also* ◄—*faiTh reversed.*

From the start, they've been defensive. And nothing you have done or said has convinced them otherwise. By the time it's all over, you will have withstood a battle of wills.

ϟ Ⓢ

Sun & Stars

UNDERNEATH & ON THE SURFACE—They want you to be happy. So let's see those pearly bright whites of yours . . . and that twinkle in your eye—at least once in a while. Lighten up. Be happy. *See also* ►—*fAte and* ◄—*fAte reversed.*

From the start, it's been in the stars. Along the way, all you've had to do is monitor the progressive developments. And by the end, it will all turn out the way it should . . . and that's pretty much the way it already is.

↑ Ⓣ

Triumph

UNDERNEATH—They want you to be a winner. So listen to your tutor, mentor, coach, or drill sergeant. Take orders. Accept criticism. Work hard at your games. Be all that you can be. *See also* ◄—*Reality.*

From the start, you have been slugging it out together. And you've been through a lot of stuff together. By the time it's all behind you, you will have a few battle scars to show . . . and a helluva story to tell.

↓ Ⓘ

Triumph reversed

ON THE SURFACE—They feel defeated. Was it something you did? Or something you can still do to make things right. Either lend a helping hand, or get the hell out. *See also* ◄—*Reality reversed.*

At the start, you were teammates. But then you became brothers in arms. And by the time it is all behind you, you will have come through the war together.

211

Birth

UNDERNEATH—They want to be your mommy and daddy. But you're getting to be a big child now. And the time will surely come when these apron strings—or is it a copper cable?—must be cut. *See also* **<**—*Karma.*

At the start, you looked up to them. And they looked out for you. But by the time it is all over, you will have taken your inheritance and gone out to seek your own fortune.

Birth reversed

ON THE SURFACE—They want to see you make it on your own. But sometimes they can't stop themselves from butting in. Your independent emergence is as gradual a process as birthing was. Try not to bite the hand that fed you. *See also* **>**—*Karma reversed.*

From the start you have both been evolving. And in the interim you have grown much. By the time it's all over, you will have helped to make each other someone else.

fEmale

UNDERNEATH—They think of you as a woman. And you will have to be the judge of what that means and whether it is flattery or insult. It could either mean they regard you as their equal or that they consider you their subordinate. *See also* **✕**—*Gifts.*

From the start, you shared your true feelings. And over the course of time you have given much of yourself. By the time it is all over, they will thank you for it. You might even get a little card or gift.

fEmale reversed

ON THE SURFACE—They see you as a man. But what do they mean when they slap you on the back? And does it make you feel good . . . or rather, nervous? Your instinctive reaction is the best barometer. *See also* ✖—*Gifts.*

From the start, you have communicated in body language. And what you really feel about each other has been expressed as much as said. By the end, you will have come to terms without speaking. At least that is your understanding.

⋈Ⓜ

Male

UNDERNEATH—They think of you as one of the guys. And there's not much you can do to disappoint them now that they've accepted you. As long as these are the people you want to hang out with, you're in like Flynn. *See also* ▶—*Wonder.*

At the beginning, you were just looking for someone to pal around with. But in the meantime, you hit it off. And by the end you will have become blood brothers without exchanging blood.

⋈Ⓦ

Male reversed

ON THE SURFACE—They think of you as one of the girls. So there's no use in putting on airs. They've divided up the roles and slotted you in yours . . . even if it was not exactly typecasting. *See also* ◀—*Wonder reversed.*

From the start, you've been set apart. But as a result, you've learned to stand up for your rights. And by the end, you will be able to fend for yourself without putting up your dukes.

▶Ⓛ

Love

UNDERNEATH—They love you . . . in the best way. And it shows. So never doubt these feelings. A love like this is unqualified . . . and very rare. Whatever you do, don't take it for granted. *See also* Ⲛ—*Hail.*

At the start, it was love at first sight. And it's only gotten better and better and better and better. It will be no different by the end.

Love reversed

ON THE SURFACE—They may not always seem to love you. But you can count on the fact that they feel a certain fondness for you. Love is gentle sometimes. And sometimes it's tough. But this time it's mostly bluff. *See also* **N**—*Hail.*

From the start, you've had your differences. And though Lord knows you've tried, it hasn't always been a bed of roses. In the end, love will have had its chance to conquer all.

beING

UNDERNEATH & ON THE SURFACE—They want you . . . in the best way . . . in the worst way . . . in every which way, including loose. And mark my words: You will surely have your bed, bath, and breakfast together yet. *See also* **✦**—*Need.*

From the start, it was a physical thing. You had a few laughs along the way. You've shared a lot. And by the end, you'll have something to talk about in your old age.

hOme

UNDERNEATH—They want you to feel at home. So feel free to pick up the TV remote and help yourself to whatever's in the fridge. Just clean up after yourself and turn the lights off when you're done. *See also* **|** —*Ice.*

You've known each other from the start. As a result, you know each other inside out. One thing's for certain: By the time it's all over, you will have come through it all together.

❤ ⓞ

hOme reversed

ON THE SURFACE—They want you to move on. So it looks to me like you've overextended your welcome, and it's time to head 'em up and move 'em out. Oh well, it was good while it lasted. *See also* **I** —*Ice.*

You've lived under the same roof, eaten at the same table, maybe even slept in the same bed. It was an experience, to be sure. And by the end, you will have developed a better idea of what you want in a roommate.

✖ ⓓ ⓞ

Destiny

UNDERNEATH & ON THE SURFACE—They like you just the way you are. So don't feel as if you have to change a bloody thing. Everything—and everybody—in this scene is A-OK. Let's try to keep it that way. *See also* ❖—*Year.*

From the start, the ending was known. In the middle the fairy tale unfolded. And in the end, they lived happily ever after.

ⵔ

weird

UNDERNEATH & ON THE SURFACE—They don't know what they want. So there's not much you can do to make them happy. So be it. Do the best you can.

From the start, it's all been up in the air. And how it all turns out, nobody, but nobody, knows.

EXTRA CREDIT

Friends forever? To find out if the two of you will have a long and mutually beneficial relationship, mix up all your Runes. Picture the other person in your mind and ask: **Are we friends forever?** Draw your fingers through your Runes and draw five, one at a time. Place them in the same "Thor's Cross" layout we used in Reading #14's Extra Credit section. . . .

Note whether each Rune is upright or reversed. Then look it up in this Reading's Answer section. For Runes 1 through 4, just read the *italic* portion of the answer. But for Rune 5 read the complete text. (You can also follow the "See Also" reference for Rune 5, if you like. Read the complete answer for that Rune as well.) Each Rune will reveal a little more of the picture, until, by the end, you will know the answer for yourself.

EXTRA, EXTRA CREDIT!

To throw your cares to the Runes. If something's got you down, cheer up by consulting your Runes. With your cares in mind, mix up your Runes and say the magic words **Double, double, take my trouble.** Draw the Rune that comes first to your hand. Turn it over face-up in front of you. Note whether it is upside down, then look it up in the Quick Reference Guide's Master Answer section. Read the whole answer and see what pops out at you.

Go on to the next Reading whenever you are ready to continue.

Reading #16

WHAT DO I NEED TO WATCH OUT FOR?
(Truth or Dare)

In this Reading you will use your Runes in order to spot your rivals,
identify your enemies, and avoid your foes. Or, for a fun diversion,
this Reading can also be used to play a round of Truth or Dare, in
which your Runes will ask you the questions.

ᛋᛋᛋ

RUNE TOOLS

Each Rune not only has a companion and an equal, but it also has
an opposite . . . a Rune that serves as its rival or nemesis. We used
these pairs in Reading #13 to get your forecast for the year.

PAIRS	RUNES		TILES	
1.	ᚠ	ᛝ	Ⓕ	Ⓓ
2.	ᚢ	ᛜ	Ⓤ	Ⓞ
3.	ᚦ	ᛨ	Ⓣⓗ	Ⓧ
4.	ᚨ	ᛚ	Ⓐ	Ⓛ
5.	ᚱ	ᛗ	Ⓡ	Ⓜ
6.	ᚲ	ᛖ	ⒸⓀ Ⓠ	Ⓔ
7.	ᚷ	ᛒ	Ⓖ	Ⓑ

217

PAIRS	RUNES		TILES		
8.	ᚠ	ᛏ	Ⓥ	Ⓦ	Ⓣ
9.	ᚺ	ᛉ	Ⓗ	Ⓢ	
10.	✝	ᛉ	Ⓝ	Ⓩ	
11.	ᛁ	ᛕ	Ⓘ	Ⓟ	
12.	ᛦ	ᛒ	Ⓨ	Ⓙ	Ⓔ

These Runic opposites will figure into the Reading you are about to do. When you draw one Rune, you will also be selecting its opposite too.

HOW TO

To find out who your challengers are . . .

1 Divide your Runes into two piles, exactly like you did in Reading #13. One pile will have the first 12 Runes (ᚠᚢᚦᚨᚱᚲᚷᚹᚺᚾᛁᛃ), and the second pile will have the last 12 Runes (ᛇᛈᛉᛋᛏᛒᛖᛗᛚᛜᛟᛞ). Place the Blank Rune in the pile of your choice.

Alphabet tile users, you know what to do. Just consult the chart in the Tools section to separate out your letters.

2 Mix up both piles of Runes separately. Think of the person or situation that you want to know about. Ask your question, **What do I need to watch out for?** with regard to this relationship? this situation? this prospect? **What opposes me?** my plans? my aspirations? Reach into one of the piles (it's your call as to which) and draw the Rune that tries to get away from you. Then turn to the second pile. Think of your question again and draw another skittish Rune.

> ## Scratch Pad
>
> *Jot down your Runes here.*

3   Look up each of your Runes, upright or reversed, in this Reading's Answer section. The text for each of your Runes includes a section on the Rune itself, as well as its opposite. Read <u>both</u> sections to get your whole answer.

For this part of the Reading, you can ignore the TRUTH and DARE sections included with the answers. But check out the Extra Credit section if you'd like to play that game with friends.

THE ANSWERS

The answers appear in the traditional order of the Runes. Reversed Runes immediately follow their upright counterparts (✖, ᚺ, ✛, ᛁ, ◇, ↓, ⚡, ⊠, ᛉ, and ☐ have no reversals).

F U Th A R K G W H N I Y Ê P Z S T B E M L X O D

ᚠ ᚢ ᚦ ᚠᚱ ᚲ ᚷ ᚹ ᚺ ᛁ ᛁ ◇ ᛃ ᛈ ᛉ ᛏ ᛒ ᛖ ᛗ ᛚ ⊠ ᛟ ᛞ

☐ **The Blank Rune appears last.**   K=C & Q; W=V; Y=J

ᚠ Ⓕ

Fortune

Beware of fortune hunters, gold diggers, and city slickers of all classes and kinds. Suspect a get-rich-quick scheme. And review all papers before you sign. *Opposite Rune:* **ᛝ**—*Destiny.* On the other hand, you're sensible enough to know the difference between a faker and the real McCoy. You never have to let yourself get suckered into anything . . . even in the big city.

TRUTH—*What's the last thing you took from a hotel?*
DARE—*Flash us the cash in your wallet.*

ᚠ Ⓕ

Fortune reversed

There are foul scoundrels in this world. Cheats. Pickpockets. Hucksters. Doctors. Lawyers. Merchants. Thieves. It seems like someone is always after your hard-earned cash. *Opposite Rune:* **ᛝ**—*Destiny.* On the other hand, you know how to look over your shoulder and out for your hip pocket. Barter down the sticker price. Ask for a discount.

TRUTH—*When's the last time you cheated someone?*
DARE—*Rip off one item of clothing.*

ᚢ Ⓤ

lUck

Be wary of your jinx . . . the thing that interrupts and distracts you, reduces your confidence, and throws you off your game. But know this: It's mostly a "mental thing" with you and not the fault of another person. *Opposite Rune:* **ᛉ**—*hOme.* But on the other hand, it's lucky you've got lots of furniture to knock on. Now, pick up the blocks, before somebody stumbles on them.

TRUTH—*When's the last time you got lucky?*
DARE—*Show us your good-luck charm.*

ↆ Ⓝ

lUck reversed

Oh, lackaday! It's just your luck! (Boy, you really know how to pick 'em.) Beware the same trap you've fallen into once. Try not to make the same mistakes twice. *Opposite Rune:* ✖—*hOme reversed.* But on the other hand, you could always click your heals thrice, Dorothy . . . if you don't want to wake up back in the Land of Oz.

TRUTH—*Are you luckier at love or cards?*
DARE—*Say "triskaidekaphobia" three times fast.*

ᚠ Ⓣⱨ

faiTh

Be wary of the ideas you buy into and off on. The tenets you sub-scribe to and the parables you preach color your entire view of real-ity . . . in black and white. *Opposite Rune:* ✖—*beING.* But on the other hand, you need to accept a few ground rules or you'll never get anything accomplished. All things in moderation, my friend. And even then, try not to get caught.

TRUTH—*When's the last time you went to church?*
DARE—*Lead us in a prayer.*

◀ Ⓣⱨ

faiTh reversed

Beware the charlatan, hypocrite, and official censor. Beware those who try to hoodwink you. And especially be wary of those who want to tell you what you should not read . . . or listen to on the head-phones. *Opposite Rune:* ✖—*beING reversed.* But on the other hand, if you're looking for the good stuff, just follow the warning labels. And if you want parental guidance, read them.

TRUTH—*When's the last time you did "the work of the devil"?*
DARE—*Say, "Madam I'm Adam" backwards.*

ᚠ Ⓐ

fAte

Beware those who tell you to stay in your place. There is no reason to ever be resigned about your lot in life. For the course is ever up and out. And you can't get there from here by standing still. *Opposite Rune:* ᚱ —*Love.* But on the other hand, if you like the status quo, there's no rule that says you have to change a bloomin' thing.

TRUTH—*What did you want to be when you grew up?*
DARE—*Kiss somebody's foot.*

ᚴ Ⓥ

fAte reversed

Beware those who try to steer you in the direction they want to go. Distrust speeches full of platitudes, slogans, moral judgments, and anything that smacks of "them" versus "us." *Opposite Rune:* ᚴ —*Love reversed.* But on the other hand, if you're no longer answering their needs, you'll be the first to know. And you can always tell them where to get off.

TRUTH—*Who did you vote for last time?*
DARE—*Do your imitation of the president.*

ᚱ Ⓡ

Reality

Beware those who market the truth. Watch out for fad diets, pop seminars, and (yikes!) "ten-minute" books. Nobody has <u>the</u> answer . . . at least not yours. *Opposite Rune:* ᛗ —*Male.* But on the other hand, you know how to pick and choose what you want to go after. You know how to cut and paste ideas together. And you know how to run it all through your computer.

TRUTH—*What's the corny motto you live by?*
DARE—*Show us the labels on your garment.*

ʁↄ

Reality reversed

Beware those who have a distorted view of reality, a limited range of experience, or a low tolerance for variation. The Universe is not homogeneous. *Opposite Rune:* ᛘ—*Male reversed.* But on the other hand, you know when the shoes you walk in are too narrow or too short. You even know how to kick them off and go barefoot.

TRUTH—Are you more afraid of failure or success?
DARE—Make a wish out loud for us.

ᚲↄↄ ᛘↄ

Course, Quest, Karma

Beware the guru, the mystic, the preacher, the teacher, and all those who claim to be enlightened. Some may be, but most are not. And no one set of ideals was ever meant to apply to everyone. *Opposite Rune:* ᛉ—*fEmale.* But on the other hand, you know how to take things with a grain of salt, a pinch of sugar, and a spoonful of Bismol.

TRUTH—Where do you want to be in three years?
DARE—Show us your photo ID.

ᚳↄↄↄ

Course, Quest, Karma reversed

Beware the prophets of doom, those who read bad signs into everything, and anyone who makes a living from pandering gloom. Even if the end <u>is</u> coming, no one has successfully predicted it yet. *Opposite Rune:* ᛦ—*fEmale reversed.* But on the other hand, I suppose it never hurts to be too careful, especially when it comes to plotting your own future.

TRUTH—When's the last time you got spooked?
DARE—Hug someone of your own gender.

✖ ⓖ ⓖ

Gifts

Beware Greeks bearing gifts, Trojan horses, subtle bribes, and any-thing that has had the price tag removed. Just because the thought counts doesn't mean it's a good omen. *Opposite Runes:* ᛒ *and* ᛤ—*Birth and reBirth.* But on the other hand, you can always decline what you cannot accept. You can always return what doesn't fit.

TRUTH—*What was the best gift you ever got?*
DARE—*Give us each a dollar.*

ᚠ Ⓥ ⓦ

Wonder

Be wary of both pessimists <u>and</u> optimists. The glass is hardly ever exactly half-empty or half-full. Our eyes play tricks on us. Or is it our own minds that are warped? *Opposite Rune:* ↑—*Triumph.* But on the other hand, you know Attitude can make a difference. And you sure know how to come to attention when The Brass pass by for proper inspection.

TRUTH—*Who's your favorite comedian?*
DARE—*Tell us your worst joke.*

ᛤ Ⓐ ⓜ

Wonder reversed

Beware those who claim everything is hunky-dory, peachy-keen, or just plain perfect. Nine times out of ten, they are being facetious. The correct response is, yeah, sure. *Opposite Rune:* ↓—*Triumph reversed.* But on the other hand, you know a limp noodle when you see it. The best way to test spaghetti is to throw it for a loop.

TRUTH—*What's your favorite pickup line?*
DARE—*Walk a straight line for us.*

ᚺ Ⓗ

Hail

Be wary of the weather forecaster, the false alarmist, and anyone else who cries wolf. Watch out too for equally fair-weathered friends who think you'll forget what you said to them yesterday. *Opposite Rune:* ᛋ—*Sun & Stars.* But on the other hand, all you have to do is look out the window to see what's really going on . . . even if you have to crane your neck.

TRUTH—*What was your last fight about?*
DARE—*Show us one of your scars.*

ᚾ Ⓝ

Need

Beware the whiner and the complainer. But most of all, be wary of the manipulator. Someone is trying to win you over. And they really know how to milk you out of your sympathy vote. *Opposite Rune:* ᛏ *and* ᚼ—*reSIStance.* But on the other hand, you still know how to say no, don't you? All you have to do is draw a line in the sand. Or better still, how about a great big circle?

TRUTH—*Who was the last person you gave your favors to?*
DARE—*Kvetch for us.*

ᛁ Ⓘ

Ice

Beware a slippery character. Some are coldhearted and ruthless beneath their high-gloss exteriors and rain-resistant paint. Watch out for carefully crafted appearances . . . and disappearances. *Opposite Rune:* ᚴ *and* ᛈ—*hoPes.* But on the other hand, you can always hold out hope—and I know you will—that this magical dragon is for real.

TRUTH—*What's the last book you read?*
DARE—*Show us the roots of your hair.*

◇ ◇ Ⓨ Ⓐ Ⓙ ⲅ

Year

Beware the Ides of March, the 29th of February, and all Fridays the 13th. But moreover, watch out for the 12th of Never and anyone who tells you how good it's going to be . . . tomorrow. *Opposite Rune:* ↑—*hElp*. But on the other hand, you've got nothing to worry about but fear itself. Let each day run out its course.

TRUTH—*What was your New Year's resolution?*
DARE—*Show us something that has your birth date on it.*

↑ Ⓔ Ⓔ

hElp

Be wary of those who profess to be concerned about your safety. I'm sure they have no other reason to want you strapped in your chair. Still, it never hurts to go into a cage cautiously. *Opposite Rune:* ◇—*Year*. But on the other hand, you don't want to become a New Year's Eve statistic either. Make a resolution to buckle up, even though it *is* the law.

TRUTH—*What do you do that you really "shouldn't"?*
DARE—*Hand over your equivalent of "cigarettes."*

Ⓚ Ⓟ

hoPe

Be wary of the Runester (yikes!), the fortuneteller, and anyone who attempts to determine your destiny by drawing numbers from a hat. Take what you need and leave the rest. *Opposite Rune:* Ⓘ—*Ice*. But on the other hand, sometimes it only takes a word or two to lock you in on something you knew anyway. If the shoe fits . . .

TRUTH—*What would you do if you won the lottery?*
DARE—*Tell us your lucky number.*

Ⓝ Ⓓ

hoPe reversed

Beware the cardsharp, the croupier, the bookie, and your State Lottery Commission. Someone wants to sucker you into supporting your favorite local charity. And nobody's getting a better education than you. *Opposite Rune:* ❘ —*Ice.* But on the other hand, it's something that you were going to do anyway. So you might as well go for your birth date, straight, cornered, and boxed.

TRUTH—*Have you ever called one of those 1-900 numbers?*
DARE—*Show us the palms of your hands.*

ᛜ Ⓩ

reSIStance

Beware the witch hunter, the vampire slayer, and any crusader hiding behind a loaded word. Someone wants to point the finger and place the blame. And I hope it's not at you. *Opposite Rune:* ᛏ—*Need.* But on the other hand, you don't have to be burned at the stake to get the point. I guess you'll either have to shape up or ship out.

TRUTH—*The last time you called in sick, were you?*
DARE—*Point the finger at someone.*

ᛘ Ⓩ

reSIStance reversed

Beware the dietary expert, the aerobics instructor, the dental hygienist, and anyone else who thinks the most important thing to do in life is floss the teeth. What about productivity? *Opposite Rune:* ᛏ—*Need.* But on the other hand, you wouldn't want to get gingivitis. And it never hurts to keep your bases covered, even if it does eat up your time.

TRUTH—*What favorite food have you given up?*
DARE—*Flex your muscles for us.*

ᛋ Ⓢ

Sun & Stars

Beware the superstar, the rising star, those who are larger than life, and those who are starry-eyed. They start to think they know everything. And worse, some start to act like it. *Opposite Rune:* ᚺ—*Hail.*

But on the other hand, you know where to buy a bag full of tomatoes. And it looks to me like you've got quite an arm on you.

TRUTH—*Whom do you admire most, and why?*
DARE—*Moon us.*

↑ Ⓣ

Triumph

Beware the soldier on furlough, the sailor on leave, the pilot on off-duty maneuvers, and anything else that resembles a ball on the rebound. There's not only a score to be kept here, but one to be settled. *Opposite Rune:* ▶—*Wonder.* But on the other hand, what's life without a couple of laughs? *From what I hear, your ship's already put in.*

TRUTH—*Are you better at all-nighters or one-nighters?*
DARE—*Show us your tattoo. (I'll settle for a birthmark.)*

↓ Ⓣ

Triumph reversed

Beware the sore loser, the poor sport, and anybody else who threatens to get back at you someday. Revenge, they say, is sweet . . . but it's better known for its sour aftertaste. *Opposite Rune:* ◀—*Wonder reversed.*   And on the other hand, it all comes back around . . . and around . . . and around. Someone's got to end this feud. It might as well be you.

TRUTH—*What's your biggest regret?*
DARE—*Pout for us.*

▶ Ⓑ

Birth

Beware the childish behavior of others. For though we are all grown-ups here, sometimes you couldn't tell it. Beneath the surface, someone is playing an ancient game with you. *Opposite Rune:* ✖—*Gifts.* But on the other hand, you remember the rules, don't you? If the ball's in your court, you better either bat it back or lose a point.

TRUTH—*What were you like as a child?*
DARE—*Show us the photo you carry of someone else.*

◀ ⑨

Birth reversed

Beware your own temper tantrums, growth spurts, and emotional outbursts. I know you can't help saying what you think sometimes. But what you blurt out at these moments is not necessarily true of how you feel in general. *Opposite Rune:* ✖—*Gifts.* But on the other hand, it's probably just something hormonal. And if you watch out for it, you can head it off.

TRUTH—*What kind of birth control do you prefer?*
DARE—*If you've got a condom on you, let's see what kind it is.*

M Ⓔ

fEmale

Beware the woman in your life? Perhaps it's that simple. But I'll bet it's something deeper. And it probably has as much or more to do with you than it does with her. *Opposite Rune:* ◀—*Karma.* But on the other hand, what I'm talking about is already obvious to you. All that's left is for you to see the light for yourself.

TRUTH—*What's something your mother always warned you about?*
DARE—*Imitate your mom for us.*

W Ⓔ

fEmale reversed

Beware the man in your life. (If you need to, you'll know who I mean.) Or else, it must be the man in you that is to blame. And if you don't know him by now, you should get to. *Opposite Rune:* ▶—*Karma reversed.* But on the other hand, what you don't know won't always hurt you. It is sometimes safer to leave well enough alone than to inquire too deeply.

TRUTH—*What's the last nice thing you did for your dad?*
DARE—*Imitate your old man for us.*

ᛗ Ⓜ

Male

Beware the guys in the band, the guys on the street, the guys in the back row. . . . The point is, there's more than one person you need to watch out for. It's when they get together that they cause you the most trouble. *Opposite Rune:* ᚱ—*Reality*. But on the other hand, you can always avoid them if you must. And if they trail along after you, you can ditch them.

TRUTH—*What's your favorite band of all time?*
DARE—*Sing a few bars of your favorite song.*

ᛗ Ⓦ

Male reversed

It's the peer pressure you want to watch out for. Just because your friends go cold turkey, does that mean you have to, too? Don't jump off any bridges just because they do. *Opposite Rune:* ᚱ—*Reality reversed*. But on the other hand, don't let others brainwash you into being a Goody Two-shoes, either.

TRUTH—*What's the worst dare you ever took?*
DARE—*Eat three crackers and give us your best wolf whistle.*

ᛚ Ⓛ

Love

Beware the love of your life—and I'm not necessarily talking about a person here. It's what you love above all else that needs to be managed. The Runes are telling you to get your priorities in order. *Opposite Rune:* ᚠ—*fAte*. But on the other hand, maybe you're already doing what you're supposed to do, even if it leaves no time for much of anything else.

TRUTH—*How many hours did you work last week?*
DARE—*Kiss the person next to you on the lips.*

230

◀ ⑦

Love reversed

Beware an estranged lover, a rejected suitor, or a jilted friend. Though you may never see them again, they have a way of creeping back into your thoughts. *Opposite Rune:* ◀—*fAte reversed.* But on the other hand, you needed to learn something from it anyway. You might as well let it stew, until it's all dissolved.

TRUTH—*How many lovers have you had?*
DARE—*Show us how you eat a banana.*

❋ Ⓧ

beING

Beware the brief affair, the one-night stand, the casual encounter . . . the midlife fling. These things have a way of being more trouble than they're worth. *Opposite Rune:* ▶ *and* ◀—*Wonders.* But on the other hand, since you're going to do it anyway—make sure you use protection, for your sake as well as that of the innocent.

TRUTH—*When's the last time you faked it?*
DARE—*Rub your head, pat your tummy, and stomp your foot.*

❖ ⊙

hOme

Beware the money pit, the landlord, the builder, the real estate agent, the mortgage company, and—did I leave anybody out?—oh yeah, the repairperson. *Opposite Rune:* ∪—*lUck.* But on the other hand, you can always hold it together with duct tape until you can afford the repairs. These days, it's all just made of plastic anyway.

TRUTH—*How much does your place set you back?*
DARE—*Fall backwards—we'll catch you.*

hOme reversed

Beware the broken home; the "home wrecker"; the city, state, and county officials; the tax collector; and anybody else who wants to put a lien on your estate. *Opposite Rune:* **Π**—*lUck reversed.* But on the other hand, you aren't going to take this lying down, are you? If it was worth having in the first place, it's worth fighting for now.

TRUTH—*Did you ever run away from home, and why?*
DARE—*Let the person to your left frisk you.*

Destiny

Be wary of lingering on the things that are done and over with. But also be wary of turning your back on your own past. If it's water under the bridge, let it go. *Opposite Rune:* **F** *and* **⊿**—*Fortunes.* But on the other hand, there is as much to be learned from failure as there is from success. You can blot out the details if you wish, but don't forget the point.

TRUTH—*What would you change about your life?*
DARE—*Trade an item of clothing with someone.*

weird

Beware! It's a big world out there, full of many possibilities and pitfalls. Some say, whatever can go wrong will. But that's only the half of it. On the other hand . . . what is meant to go *right* will, too.

TRUTH—*Did you ever have a wish come true?*
DARE—*Pick another Rune if you double-dog dare (but you <u>must</u> tell the truth it asks).*

EXTRA CREDIT

To play Truth or Dare. Invite a few friends over to "do Runes." What the heck, make it a theme party . . . something Celtic or

Viking would be good. (I'll wear my hooded robe.) Anyway, once everybody's ready to begin . . . just mix up your Runes and say, "Truth or Dare." Reach into your Rune bag and grab the first two that you get. Or take a handful of Runes, toss them on the floor, and reach out and grab the first two you come in contact with. Place them in front of you, upright or reversed. . . .

1   **2**

Truth   **Dare**

Now turn to this Reading's Answer section. Find your first Rune, and read the TRUTH that it asks for. Then look up your second Rune to learn the DARE you can opt for if the truth is just too embarrassing to tell. Take your turn by telling the TRUTH or taking the DARE. Then pass the bag of Runes on to the next person. Appoint a designated driver.

EXTRA, EXTRA CREDIT!

For a funky experience. Don't ask any question at all. Just mix up all your Runes. Say, **Fe, Fi, Fo, Fum**, and draw three Runes just as fast as you can get hold of them. . . .

Reading: **1**   **2**   **3**
            #16   #15   #14

Look up your Runes, as indicated, in Readings #16, #15, and #14. And don't be a bit surprised if a question that's been on your mind gets answered in the process. For more group fun, check out the other party games listed in the index. Or play a game of Scrabble®.

Go on to the next Reading whenever you are ready to continue.

Reading #17

TELL ME A BEDTIME STORY
(Lay me odds)

In this Reading, the Runes are going tell you a little story that will pertain to your life and give you something to think about. Or you can use this Reading to draw or cast Runes in order to calculate the odds that anything you'd like to bet on will take place as planned.

↑ ↑ ↑

RUNE TOOLS

The Runes of the Elder Futhark can be thought of as three groups (or tiers) of eight Runes each, starting with the first Rune (**F**), the ninth Rune (**H**), and the 17th Rune (**T**). Reading from left to right . . .

	1	2	3	4	5	6	7	8
1	F	U	Þ	F	R	<	X	P
2	H	ᛏ	I	ᛋ	ᛃ	K	Y	S
3	T	B	M	M	ᛚ	ᛜ	ᛟ	M

For alphabet-tile users . . .

	1	2	3	4	5	6	7	8
1	F	U	Th	A	R	K	G	W
2	H	N	I	Y	E	P	Z	S
3	T	B	E	M	L	X	O	D

K = C Q   W = V   Y = J

234

In this Reading we will be working with all three tiers of Runes, aided by some pictures that illustrate their meanings.[1]

HOW TO

To hear your story . . .

1   Sort your Runes into three piles: 1) ᚠ ᚢ ᚦ ᚨ ᚱ ᚲ ᚷ ᚹ, 2) ᚺ ᚾ ᛁ ᛃ ᛇ ᛈ ᛉ ᛊ,   and 3) ᛏ ᛒ ᛖ ᛗ ᛚ ᛜ ᛟ ᛞ. Place the Blank Rune in the pile of your choice. Or, to use alphabet tiles, use the chart in the Tools section to identify the letters you need in each pile.

2   Now mix up your Runes—one pile at a time—while you think of your question: **Tell me a tale about _____.** my work life. my love life. a past life. **Tell me a tale about my relationship with _____.** my job with _____. Or simply, **Tell me a story.**

3   Reach into the first pile and pick the Rune that comes into your hand. Place it Rune side up in front of you. Then repeat your question, reach into the second pile of Runes, and draw the second. Place it to the right of the first. Finally, repeat your question again, reach into the third pile of Runes, and draw another Rune.

Scratch Pad

Jot down your Runes here.

---

[1] My great thanks to Pittsburgh artist William B. Cox for his faithful and inspired rendering of the Runes. ᛉ ᛜ ᛉ

Look up your first Rune in <u>this</u> Reading's Answer section. Look up the second in the <u>next</u> Reading's Answer section (Reading #18). And look up the last Rune in Reading #19.

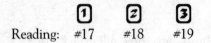

Reading: #17   #18   #19

To consider your answer, look first at the artist's rendering of your Rune and then read the brief story beside it. For additional clues to the meaning, consult the keywords for your Rune (upright or reversed). Think about it all for a minute, especially the picture. Then read between the lines.[2]

THE ANSWERS

The answers appear in the traditional order of the Runes. Reversed Runes are covered under their upright counterparts. (Though **✕**, **H**, **✝**, **❘**, **◇**, **↗**, **S**, **✵**, **M**, and **☐** typically have no reversals, reversed meanings have been included for each of the drawings, since if you were using these drawings as playing cards, each could "fall" upside down.)

Reading #17	F	U	Th	A	R	K	G	W	☐
Reading #18	H	N	I	Y	Ê	P	Z	S	☐
Reading #19	T	B	E	M	L	X	O	D	☐

K=C & Q; W=V; Y=J

Reading #17	ᚠ	ᚢ	ᚦ	ᚨ	ᚱ	ᚲ	ᚷ	ᚹ	☐
Reading #18	ᚺ	ᚾ	ᛁ	ᛃ	ᛇ	ᛈ	ᛉ	ᛊ	☐
Reading #19	ᛏ	ᛒ	ᛖ	ᛗ	ᛚ	ᛜ	ᛟ	ᛞ	☐

[2] The basic format for this Answer set is borrowed from actress, tarot expert, and author Eden Grey, whose work has influenced me greatly. Readings #17, #18, and #19 are graciously dedicated to her.

FORTUNE

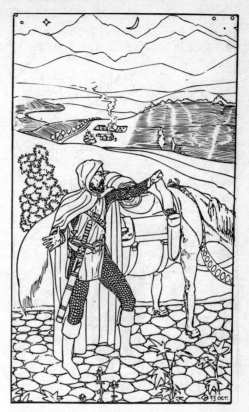

Once upon a time, there was a fellow who had everything going for him: a fine set of wheels, great threads, plenty of bread, and a warm bed. The world lay at his feet. He wanted to see it all, do it all, have it all, be it all, go for it all. So one day he packed his gear and went to seek his fortune—thus risking everything.

Money matters are of utmost importance. **Keywords. Upright:** Land, real estate, property. Birthright, inheritance, capital gains. Count your assets. **Reversed:** Lack of means. Shortage of funds. Rents, loans, and interest due. Disinheritance. Sale of personal property. Compute your net worth.

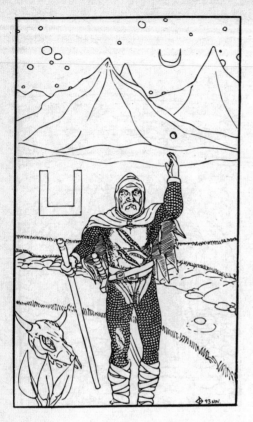

l**U**ck

Once upon a time, there was a fellow who fought hard for everything he had coming and worked hard for everything he got. Yet if you asked him, he'd tell you it was not entirely his own doing and that luck had played its part. One day, battle-worn and separated from his party, he yet had cause to feel that luck was on his side. Tossing a piece of silver to the moon, he made his wish for luck to abide.

Luck is on your side. **Keywords.** **Upright:** Good luck. Safe journey. Good health. Long life. Sure deliverance. Make a wish upon a star. **Reversed:** A change in luck. A lucky break. Break a leg. Keep your fingers crossed.

FAITH

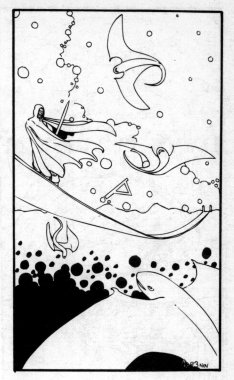

Once upon a time, there was a fellow who believed everything they said in church. He believed that all creation was a battle between good and evil. And so he went forth in faith to wage his holy war against the dark powers. But as it turned out, the only demons he ever really encountered were those inside himself. And it was like dueling with shadows.

You need to believe. **Keywords. Upright:** Belief in God, motherhood, and apple pie. Faith. Hope. Trust. Will. A religious experience. **Reversed:** Belief in yourself. High spirits. The power of positive thinking. Resolve. Resolution. A spiritual experience. Freedom from guilt.

fATE

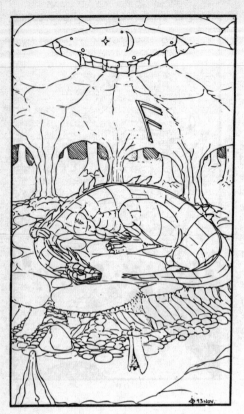

Once upon a time, there was a fellow who went looking for himself. He traveled far and wide in the process, saw many strange things, heard many a tale, and escaped numberless perils. Not knowing what he was looking for, it took him a while to realize his fate was not something that lay in wait for him. But rather, he was already its living proof.

Work with what you've got. **Keywords. Upright:** External forces and conditions. Circumstances. Environmental influences. Live within your means. **Reversed:** Internal forces. Reaction to conditions, circumstances. Don't let it get to you. Don't let it get you down.

Ｒ

REALITY

Once upon a time there was a fellow who wanted to prove himself. So he put on his backpack and headed out to brave the wilderness alone. For many hot and sweaty days—and as many cold and lonely nights—he ventured forth on his own two feet, feeling rugged, independent, and free. But in the end, he tired of sleeping alone and decided to return to the real world.

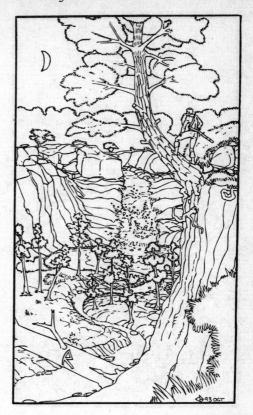

Seek and you will find. **Keywords**. **Upright:** Travel by land, water, or air. Spiritual journey. Vision quest. Get some distance to gain new insight. **Reversed:** Change of scenery. A weekend retreat or getaway. A new outlook. Enjoy a refreshing change of pace.

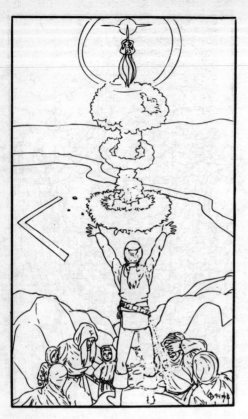

COURSE, QUEST, KARMA

Once upon a time, there was a fellow who saw something odd in the sky. And all the people took it as a sign. Thus his purpose was made known to him in a blinding flash of light and a roar of thunder. From that day forward, he had no choice but to take the role thrust upon him, be it hero, saint, or martyr. It was his calling.

The way will be revealed. **Keywords. Upright:** Enlightenment. Revelation. Inspiration. Let all mortal flesh keep silence. Look for the signs. **Reversed:** A message from heaven. The light at the end of the tunnel. Take one step at a time. Pray for a miracle. Ask for a sign.

GIFTS

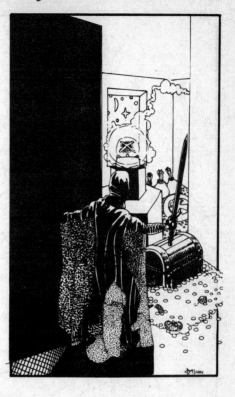

Once upon a time there was a fellow who had rare and unusual gifts, special talents, and even, some said, the Midas touch when it came to working marvels. It seemed as if he could do anything he put his mind to. It seemed as if he could snap his fingers and things would just happen. But mostly he practiced hard at it. And that's what made it seem like magic.

Make use of your gifts. **Keywords.** **Upright:** Appreciation. Mutual admiration. Craft and craftsmanship. Apply your talents, skills, and psychic abilities. **Picture Reversed:** Fantasies, illusions, and pipe dreams. Tricks and trickery. Discipline. Determination. Do it until you get it right.

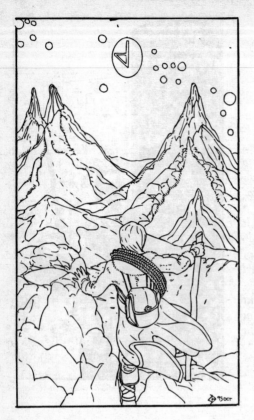

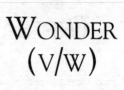

WONDER (V/W)

Once upon a time there was a fellow who climbed to the top of the mountain just because it was there. And everybody wondered what he was trying to prove. But they didn't understand. It was not for the hero's welcome on the other side—or even to get to say he had done it. Pure and simply, it was for the thrill of the moment. And wow! What a high!

Have a blast. **Keywords. Upright:** Joy. Delight in life. Bliss. A thrill a minute. Awe. Reverence. Respect. See the world through the eyes of a child. **Reversed:** A steep uphill climb. A goal in sight. Getting there is half the fun. Take time to enjoy the day.

☐

WEIRD

Once upon a time there was a fellow who had a clean slate and a box of colored chalk. But there he sat looking at the blank board. What should he draw this time? How should it start? When there are all the possibilities in the world, the hardest part is making the first choice.

Be open to the options. **Keywords. Upright:** Everything . . . nothing. Emptiness . . . fullness. The void. Clay that needs shaped. Ideas that need substance. Thoughts that need voiced. Urges that need acted upon. Strange feelings. Subconscious thoughts. Feel your way along. **Reversed:** Same as above.

EXTRA CREDIT

To calculate the odds. Mix up your Runes while you think of your question: **What are the odds I'll _____?** get that promotion? interview? offer? What are the odds we'll get together? What are the odds the house will sell this month? This method works with just about any question you can think of asking about work, love, money, or whatnot. Select two Runes and lay them side by side. Or cast a handful of Runes and pick the two that feel the most likely.

Look up your first Rune in the table in this Reading's Tools section. Jot down the number (1-8) along the top of the chart that is directly above your Rune. (The Blank Rune is worth a 9). Place a colon (:) after it. Then look up your second Rune, and jot down its number after the colon. You now have your odds.

Let's say I drew **ᚠ** and **ᚦ**. Since **ᚠ** is worth a 1 and **ᚦ** is worth a 3, my odds are 1:3 . . . or, in other words, one in three. (If your Runes turn up reversed, not to worry. They have the same number upside down as upright.)

EXTRA, EXTRA CREDIT!

To make flash cards. Here's a fun and effective way to learn your Runes. Just get yourself some poster board and cut it into 25 card-like shapes. Or use 25 3-by-5 index cards. Starting with eight cards, take a red felt-tip marker and draw one of the first eight Runes from this Reading in the center of each card, leaving one card blank. Now go back and write the Rune's name under it.[3]

You can also copy down a few keywords and phrases from this Reading's Answer section on each card. Just select the words that strike home to you and jot them down, upright meanings on the top. Turn the card around (so the Runes are upside down) and write the reversed meanings on the bottom.

To use your flash cards, just gather them together and "run through them" every night, starting with these first eight. Before you go to sleep, look at each Rune in turn, say its name, and read the keywords. You will literally learn the Runes in your sleep! And be sure to pay attention to your dreams. Turn to the Extra, Extra Credit section of Reading #18 to continue the process with the next eight Runes.

Go on to the next Reading whenever you are ready to continue.

---

[3] You can also add numbers. But you will probably want to use the chart from Reading #12's Tools section, where the Runes are numbered from 1 to 25.

Reading #18

WHAT'S THE WORD?
(Run interference for me)

In this Reading you'll be using your Runes to get your watchwords for the days, weeks, months, and years ahead. Or you can also use this Reading to select a Rune that will help you remove the obstacles and barriers to your personal progress.

ᛒ ᛒ ᛒ

RUNE TOOLS

In Reading #17 we started to think of the Runes in the Elder Futhark as three groups (or tiers) of eight Runes each. In this Reading we will be working with the same three tiers again. Here's your cheat sheet . . .

As in the previous Reading, we will be using artist's renderings of the Runes to interpret the answers.

HOW TO

To get your keywords . . .

1   Separate your Runes or alphabet tiles into three piles. Put the first eight Runes in the first pile, the second eight Runes in the second pile, and the third eight in the last pile. Place the Blank Rune in the pile of your choice. Consult the chart in this Reading's Tools section if you need help.

2   Mix up each pile of Runes separately while you think of your question: **What words of advice do you have for me today?** for tomorrow? for next week? for the year ahead? Or simply, **What's the word?** on my job offer? with my affairs in general? in my relationship with so-and-so?

3   From the first pile, select the Rune that worms its way into your hand. Place it Rune side up in front of you. Then, select a Rune from the second pile, placing it next to the Rune you drew before. Finally, select a Rune from the third pile, placing it next to the other two.

Scratch Pad

Jot down your Runes here.

248

Look up your First Rune in Reading #17's Answer section. Look at the picture for your Rune and read the keywords for your upright or reversed Rune. Focus on the words that jump out at you today.

	1	2	3
Reading:	#17	#18	#19

Look up your second Rune in Reading #18. And look up your third Rune in Reading #19.

THE ANSWERS

The answers appear in the traditional order of the Runes. Reversed Runes are covered under their upright counterparts. (Though ᚷ, ᚺ, ᚾ, ᛁ, ᛃ, ᛇ, ᛊ, ᛜ, ᛞ, and □ typically have no reversals, reversed meanings have been included for each of the drawings, since if you were using these drawings as playing cards, each could "fall" upside down.)

Reading #17	F	U	Th	A	R	K	G	W	□
Reading #18	H	N	I	Y	Ê	P	Z	S	□
Reading #19	T	B	E	M	L	X	O	D	□

K=C & Q; W=V; Y=J

Reading #17	ᚠ	ᚢ	ᚦ	ᚨ	ᚱ	ᚲ	ᚷ	ᚹ	□
Reading #18	ᚺ	ᚾ	ᛁ	ᛃ	ᛇ	ᛈ	ᛉ	ᛊ	□
Reading #19	ᛏ	ᛒ	ᛖ	ᛗ	ᛚ	ᛜ	ᛟ	ᛞ	□

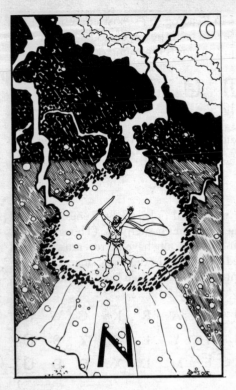

H

HAIL

It was a dark and stormy night. And at times it seemed as if Pandora's box had opened just a crack to let us glimpse God's wrath. There was thunder and lightning . . . intermittent driving rain . . . the ticking of sleet . . . the knocking of hail . . . and winds that took your breath away. And it would take a brave and clever man indeed to earn his living as a rain-maker.

Hold on to your hat. **Keywords.** **Upright:** External conditions. Forces outside your control. Hostile atmosphere. Bad vibrations. Watch for a sudden change in the weather. **Picture Reversed:** Internal conditions. Forces within your control. Take responsibility for your own actions.

NEED

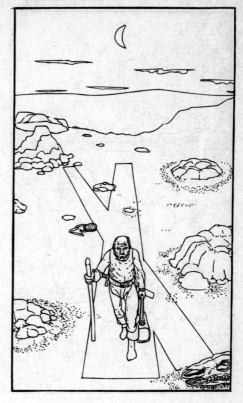

There was hardly enough of anything, except for the oppressive heat of the day and the bone-chilling cold of the night. The traveler was hungry, thirsty, tired, and dirty. And the odds against him were great. Yet, with a firm will, he trudged forward into the vast emptiness . . . wishing for salvation, needing a miracle.

Give it one more shot. **Keywords. Upright:** Want. Need. Deep do-da. Big trouble. Not enough to get by on. Less than you deserve. Keep hanging in there. **Picture Reversed:** Down on your luck. Hardly a leg to stand on. Thirsty for something. Decide what you can make do with. . . and without.

I

ICE

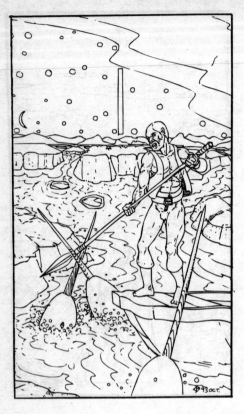

First came the frost, and with it a chill wind that cut to the quick. The sky turned black around the edges. Then came the snow . . . the freezing rain . . . and sheets of ice that stopped everything in its tracks. It felt like things were closing in from all sides. But still the brave soul fought on . . . to the bitter end.

Things are changing shape. **Keywords. Upright:** Channels closing. Restrictions, constrictions, blockages. Caught between a rock and a hard place. Think fast. Act faster. See your way around obstacles. **Picture Reversed:** Avenues opening up. Barriers melting. Build a fire under yourself.

YEAR
(Y/J)

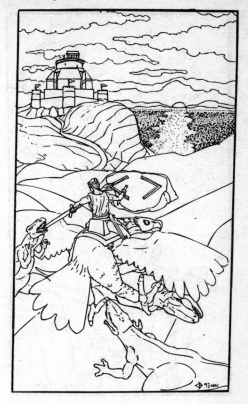

It was so close he could taste it . . . the end of the journey, the completion of the mission. All the hours of preparation and the days of working toward this goal had come—at last—into view. Just this one last deed to do. And done! The sun sank in the west. The moon rose in the east. Night fell. The time of waiting had passed slow-ly—yet quickly still. And then everything reached closure.

Timing is everything. **Keywords.** **Upright:** Fulfillment. Completion. Resolution. Climax. Safe passage. What a difference a year makes. **Picture Reversed:** Unavoidable delays. Extenuating circumstances. One last battle to endure. Hold on tight. It's only a matter of time.

hElp

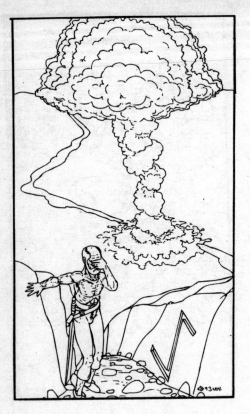

It came in a blinding flash from out of the blue, and with a rumble that shook the firm earth. The dust kicked up. The repercussion fanned out in waves. The eyewitness saw nothing but a flash. And afterwards there was nothing to be done about it, but repent. Speak no evil. Hear no evil. See no evil.

You need to save yourself. **Keywords.** **Upright:** Up to your elbows. In over your head. Out on a limb. It's time to bring in the big guns and put Plan B into effect. **Picture Reversed:** Worries and concerns. Fear. Paranoia. Deep, dark secrets. Confide only in those who can be trusted.

HOPE

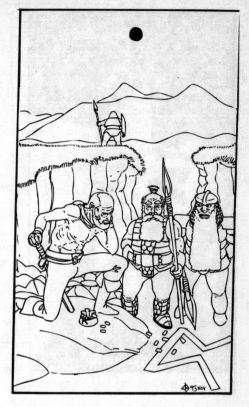

Two paths diverged . . . one way familiar, and the other completely foreign. The Runes made a favorable sound when they fell to the ground. But the signs themselves were open to interpretation. The Runester sat and pondered for the longest while . . . until, at last, he made some sense of them. And he decided down which path his destiny lay.

Give it your best shot. **Keywords. Upright:** Omens. Signs. Probabilities. Games of chance. Decisions to make. Verdicts to reach. Make up your mind. **Reversed:** Luck of the draw. Split decision. Six of one, half a dozen of the other. A mixed bag. The jury is still out. Decide for yourself.

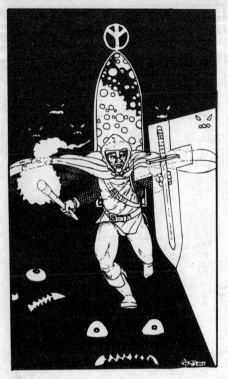

reSISTANCE (Z)

It was the witching hour, I guess. The tired pilgrim's eyes were playing tricks on him. A shadow in the corner suddenly shifted. A thump outside the window made him flinch. Suddenly it felt like eyes were watching from the shadows of the room. And with his heart pounding, he threw open the door to the closet. But the only skeletons in there were his.

You are being protected. **Keywords. Upright:** Assistance from an unseen hand. Guardian angels. Unseen forces—and counter-forces—at work. Wear your good luck charms and amulets. **Reversed:** Phantoms of the mind. Inner demons. You must confront your shadows.

Sun & Stars

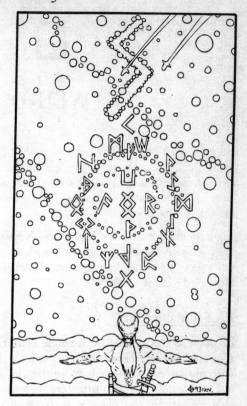

There had never been such a night. The sky seemed to go on forever. Stars, planets, smoky galaxies . . . there were even shooting stars going off like stray fireworks. It was as if the heavens had decided to dance for us in their wheel-within-their-wheel. Everything was humming along to the music of the spheres. And nothing else seemed to matter.

Things are unfolding as they should. **Keywords. Upright:** The Universe. Cosmic time. Your world. The larger purpose. The bigger picture. Look for the meaning in your life. **Picture Reversed:** Continuity. One thing leading to another. Everything in its proper time and season. Pursue your own special purpose.

O

WEIRD

Everything felt empty inside, as if the wish of the mind no longer mattered and the emotions were no longer felt. There was not so much as a butterfly in the stomach, let alone a cc of adrenaline in the blood. In that calm, quiet moment, the answer simply came. The truth was not only known . . . but accepted.

Look for unexpected developments. **Keywords. Upright:** Intuitive leap. Creative spark. Spontaneous idea. Important realization. All the pieces suddenly fit together. Eureka! You have your answer. **Reversed:** Same as above.

EXTRA CREDIT

To overcome obstacles (in a single bound). Gather all your Runes together and ask, **How can I remove the barriers to my progress?** with my career? with the lady (or the man)? as a lover? friend? parent? Or simply say, **Run interference for me.** Then select the Rune that feels right and place it in front of you. Consult the Quick Reference Guide's Master Answer section for your Rune (upright or reversed) and pay particular attention to the portion of the text on strategy. For luck, carry your Rune around in your pocket for a day or so.

EXTRA, EXTRA CREDIT!

To continue making flash cards. From the cardboard squares you cut and marked in Reading #17, pull out eight more cards. Copy down the Runes, Rune names, and keywords from this Reading's Answer section, just as you did with the first eight cards. Upright meanings go on the top. Flip your card, and write reversed meanings on the bottom.

Run through these new cards at bedtime. As you come to each, look at the Rune, recite its name, and read its meanings. Then sleep on it. Note what you wake up thinking about.

Go on to the next Reading whenever you are ready to continue.

Reading #19

WHERE WILL I BE AT THE END OF THE DAY?
(Find me love)

In this Reading you'll be using your Runes to project the outcome
you can expect from any activity, interest, or endeavor. You can
also use this Reading to draw or cast Runes in order to determine
who (or what!) the true love of your life is.

MMM

RUNE TOOLS

In interpreting your answers for this Reading, you'll continue to use
the Answer sets from Readings #17 and #18. For help in looking up
your Runes, here's a chart that shows which Runes are covered
where . . .

Reading 17:

F U Þ F R < X P
(F) (U) (Th) (A) (R) (K) (G) (W)

Reading 18:

H + I ◇ ↑ K Y S
(H) (N) (I) (Y) (E) (P) (Z) (S)

Reading 19:

↑ B M M ↑ ⋈ ⋄ ⋈
(T) (B) (E) (M) (L) (X) (O) (D)

(K) = (C) (Q)   (W) = (V)   (Y) = (J)

HOW TO

To assess the outcome of any matter that concerns you . . .

1   Gather <u>all</u> your Runes or alphabet tiles together and mix them up while you think of the matter that concerns you.

2   Ask your question: **How will this thing pay off?** our relationship pan out? this project turn out? **Where will this all get me?** Where will I wind up? **Where will I be at the end of the day?**

3   Select the three Runes that come to your fingertips and place them in front of you in a line.

Scratch Pad

Jot down your Runes here.

Use the chart in the Tools section to locate your Runes in the book. For each Rune, the chart will show you whether to look it up in Reading #17, #18, or #19. If you draw the Blank Rune, look up your answer in any of the three Readings—your choice! Or, what the 🄷 🄴 🄲 🄺, read all three and take your pick.

THE ANSWERS

The answers appear in the traditional order of the Runes. Reversed Runes are covered under their upright counterparts. (Though ✕, **H**, ✝, **I**, ◇, ✦, ⑀, ⍓, ⋈, and ⬭ typically have no reversals, reversed meanings have been included for each of the drawings, since if you were using these drawings as playing cards, each could "fall" upside down.)

Reading #17   F   U   Th   A   R   K   G   W   ⬭

Reading #18   H   N   I   Y   Ê   P   Z   S   ⬭

Reading #19   T   B   E   M   L   X   O   D   ⬭

K=C & Q; W=V; Y=J

Reading #17   ᚠ   ᚢ   ᚦ   ᚨ   ᚱ   ᚲ   ✕   ᚹ   ⬭

Reading #18   **H**   ✝   **I**   ◇   ✦   ᛲ   ⍓   ⑀   ⬭

Reading #19   ↑   ᛒ   M   ⋈   ᛚ   ⑀   ⋏   ⋈   ⬭

TRIUMPH

It was not a fair fight. The opponent was bigger and stronger and played by different rules. For a while there—amid the smoke and flames—it could have gone either way. The victor thought more quickly on his feet and threw a few luckier punches. And by the end of the day, it was you who emerged the "better man."

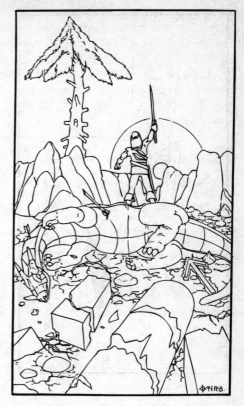

All's well that ends well. **Keywords. Upright:** Conquest. Victory. Defeat of rivals and opponents. Triumph over enemies and bad influences. Make a speech. Take a bow. **Reversed:** Self-control. Mastery over internal "demons." A winning attitude. A fighting spirit. Be noble. Be loyal.

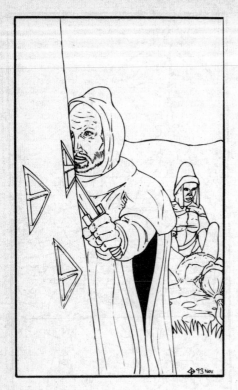

BIRTH

You labored long and hard for your deliverance. For even the most natural of transitions can be a painful experience. With help of Runes, perhaps, but certainly with aid of caring friends, you pulled through the crisis. And soon the agony was but a vague memory, overpowered with the sheer joy of having lived through it. Wow! What a ride!

You are starting all over. **Keywords. Upright:** Creativity and procreativity. Fertility. Pregnancy. Childbirth. To feel like a new person. **Reversed:** Turning point. Transition. Rite of passage. Personal transformation. Change in style. Change in looks. Change in attitude.

M

fEMALE

It was a funny feeling you had. Suddenly it was no longer your own reflection staring back at you from the mirror, the darkened windowpane, the rippling water. Suddenly your mind was somewhere else. You had an inkling. You had a kenning. Words came into your head. Events unfolded before your very eyes. And you knew the future.

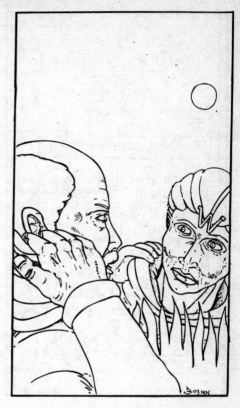

You can trust your inclinations. **Keywords. Upright:** Precognition. Vision. Gut feeling. Intuition. Sixth sense. Pick up on the things that make you tick. **Reversed:** Male and female ways. Feminine characteristics. Take your cues from the woman in your life. Look inside yourself for the answers.

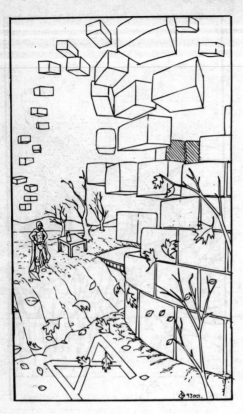

MALE

You had a dream that possessed you. And in your mind's eye, it played out again and again. You built your castles in the air. You made your plans and drew your blueprints. You plotted your next moves until, little by little, the dream took shape. At last, all the pieces had fallen into place, and you were able to cross another goal off your list.

You <u>can</u> have it your own way. ***Keywords*. Upright:** Goals. Objectives. High hopes. Big ambitions. Accomplishments. Making something out of nothing. **Reversed:** Mental tests, puzzles, problems. Build on the past. Tear things apart. Put them back together again.

LOVE

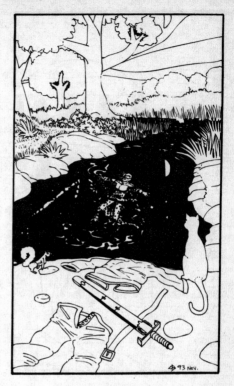

The sun was low on the horizon. And a Quarter Moon was in the sky. The pool felt welcome after the heat of the day. The pitch-blackening water closed in around your buck-naked body, hiding your private parts, and buoying up your hopes. And it felt good to be alive again, didn't it? Besides, it was plain to see you were in love.

Take time to love and be loved. **Keywords. Upright:** Lifeblood. The eternal stream. The waters of life. Go with the flow. Get into the groove. Dance to the beat. **Reversed:** Hang it all. Hang loose. Hang it out to dry. Be as innocent as on the day you were born.

beING

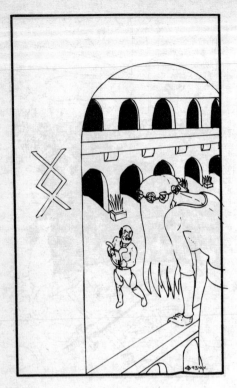

In the moonlight it was hard to tell whether he was a satyr or a suitor. But he sure did have his lines down well. She was—quite frankly—the sexiest thing he'd ever laid eyes on. It was a night to remember— the scent of the honeysuckle . . . hushed voices on the balmy air . . . and the pounding of your two thundering hearts so distant and yet so close.

If it feels good, do it. **Keywords. Upright:** Making love. Courtship. Romance. Foreplay. Commitment. To win the heart, take first things first. **Picture Reversed:** Kisses. Hugs. Sighs. The flames of passion. The depths of desire. Love the one you're with.

hOME

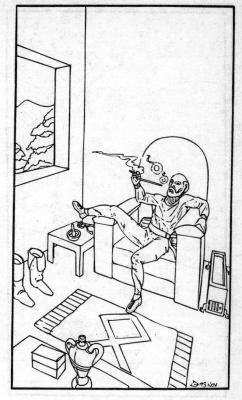

The sun was setting in shades of scarlet behind the purple hills. And the last light of day bathed the room in a low and hazy glow. All the sights and sounds of the man-made world wound down outside. The crickets and cicadas began to hum. And in the magic of that solitary moment, you got the message at last. Be it ever so humble, this is your place.

Live your own life in your own way. ***Keywords.*** **Upright:** A place of your own. Four walls. A roof over your head. A place to call home. Hang on to what you've got. **Reversed:** Invasion of privacy. Big Brother is watching. Smoke if you've got 'em—but close the blinds first.

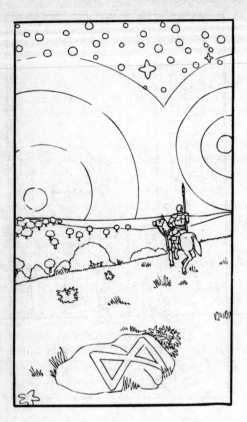

DESTINY

It was all said and done . . . done and over . . . over and gone, except for the riding off into the sunset part. Everything that happened in the past led up to this moment of conclusion. And with it came a new beginning and a chance to start all over again. Older and wiser now, you go forth. But first pause to reflect and take a deep breath.

Do what comes naturally. **Keywords. Upright:** Perfect endings. New beginnings. Completion. Resolution. A matter works itself out. Don't worry. **Picture Reversed:** Eternity. Endless possibilities. Man, woman, birth, death, infinity. Things go on and on. Be happy.

O

WEIRD

It was a dense fog that had blown in. Visibility was low. The margin for error was pretty slim. And the only way to go was to feel your way like a blind man crossing the street. The mists rolled through the looming trees. Oh Great Spirit, tell me: Are these the shadows of the things that will be? Or might they yet be changed?[1]

Dare to defy your fate. **Keywords. Upright:** A blind alley. A dead-end street. Yet . . . there is still time to change. Shape the present. Mold the future. Alter your destiny. And do it now, while you still have the chance. **Reversed:** Same as above.

EXTRA CREDIT

To find your true love. Mix up all your Runes while you think of your question: **What's the great love of my life? What love will I know? What kind of love will find me?** Or simply, **Find me love.** Draw three Runes and look them up in the Quick Reference Guide's Master Answer section.

Physical   **Emotional**   **Spiritual**

The first Rune you draw will tell you what you love to do. The second Rune will tell you what you love to feel. And the third Rune will tell you where your great happiness lies.

You can also ask about a specific person. Just say, **What kind of love will so-and-so be?** Or about a thing: **What kind of love do I feel for _____?** my work? my art? my craft? my dog? my house?

---

[1] Scrooge to the Ghost of Christmas Yet to Come. Paraphrased from Stave 4, *A Christmas Carol.* With many thanks to Charles Dickens for a most inspiring tale.

my RV? Not everything written in the Master Answer section will apply to every question. Take what you need.

EXTRA, EXTRA CREDIT!

To finish your flash cards. To complete the Rune cards you started in Reading #17, sort out the last eight cards from your deck and copy down the Runes and keywords from this Reading's Answer section. Flip them around and write the reverse meanings.

To conduct this Reading with your cards, shuffle all your cards together while you ask your question: **What will I have at the end of today?** When the cards are done (you'll just know), deal up the top three, and look them up in Readings #17, #18, or #19, as appropriate. Your new cards will work with any Reading in this book!

To continue learning your Runes at night, just flip through your cards before you go to sleep. If any Runes happen to appear in your dreams, don't forget to look them up in the Master Answer section.

Go on to the next Reading whenever you are ready to continue.

Reading #20

WHAT WILL I AMOUNT TO?
(Give me values)

In this Reading, you will literally "add up" the Runes in your name to find out what your prospects are in life and identify your strong points. You can also use this Reading to draw or cast Runes in order to think about ethical questions or moral issues.

ᛗᛗᛗ

RUNE TOOLS

Each Rune has a numerical "value" as well as a number of its own. This value can be found by simply consulting this chart . . .

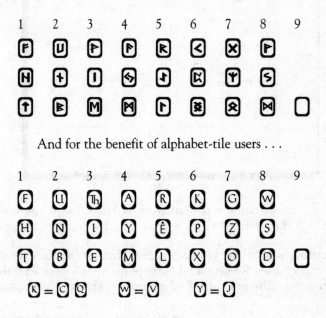

And for the benefit of alphabet-tile users . . .

Each Rune also embodies *real*—moral, ethical, and human—*values*, which you'll learn about as you do this Reading. For this purpose, we'll be working with the original Anglo-Saxon Rune names that you last used in Reading #7 or #8, depending on which course you've taken through the book.

HOW TO

To see what you'll amount to . . .

1 Go back to the How To section of Reading #5, where you wrote your family name in Runes. Copy your last name in Runes onto this Scratch Pad. Or simply translate it again . . .

Scratch Pad

Jot down your Runes here.

Use the family name you were given at birth. But if you have adopted another last name, jot it down too, for comparative purposes.

In writing your name, remember that **Th** and **-ing** have single Runes of their own. Remember that there are two E's—use **M** if the sound is long, otherwise use **↑**. And remember that apostrophes, hyphens, periods, or blank spaces also count. Add a Blank Rune to your name for each of these items that occurs.

② Now, for each and every Rune in your family name, jot down its corresponding number (1 to 9) from the table in this Reading's Tools section. For example, let's say my name is Rezak. I would jot down these Runes and numbers: R/ᚱ = <u>5</u>, E/ᛗ = <u>3</u>, Z/ᛉ = <u>7</u>, A/ᚠ = <u>4</u>, K/ᚲ = <u>6</u>.

③ Now add these numbers together. In Rezak's case: 5 + 3 + 7 + 4 + 6 = 25. Then <u>add</u> again: 2 + 5 = 7. (If you still have a number of 10 or higher at this point, add again: 1 + 0 = 1.[1]) Look up your number in the Answer section. In Rezak's case, it's number 7.

Your answer consists of the three Runes associated with your number. Read the main text, which describes your combination of Runes. Then from the list of values that follows, choose the one or two that strike home to you today.

THE ANSWERS

The Runes appear in their traditional numerical order, but they are listed in trios. Reversed Runes are listed under their upright counterparts (✗, ᚺ, ✦, ᛁ, ◇, ↑, ⟨, ✹, ᛗ, and □ have no reversals).

F	U	T	A	R	K	G	W	
H	N	I	Y	Ê	P	Z	S	
T	B	E	M	L	X	O	D	□

ᚠ	ᚢ	ᚦ	ᚠ	ᚱ	ᚲ	✗	ᚠ	
ᚺ	✦	ᛁ	◇	↑	ᚾ	ᛉ	ᛋ	
↑	ᛒ	ᛗ	ᛗ	ᛚ	✹	ᛩ	ᛗ	□

K=C & Q; W=V; Y=J

ᚠ ⓕ   ᚺ ⓗ   ↑ ⓣ

Fortune   Hail   Triumph

1 All's well that ends well, my friend . . . so your motto should be. For from your life you will savor most the moments of resolution.

[1] The method we're using here is classic Greek numerology as taught by the mathematician/philosopher Pythagoras (Sixth century B.C.).

Here is your trilogy of Runes: The **F**-Rune sees that you get the resources you need. The **H**-Rune keeps you challenged. And the **T**-Rune provides the stamina and endurance to succeed in the battles you choose to fight. You have the wherewithal to overcome the things that distract and discourage others. You have the ability to know both fame and fortune, in your own way and in your own time. You will amount to the reputation that you make for yourself. Choose your values . . .

F Ⓕ *Fehu—The cattle are numbered by the head. You place a high value on things that can be assessed, sold off, or bartered. You believe in acquiring things that add to your net worth.*

◢ Ⓕ *Fehu reversed—The cattle are branded on the rump. You value property ownership and the laws that protect it. You believe in investing in the future.*

H Ⓗ *Hail—The storm clouds gathering give fair warning. Be attentive to the signs. You value the ability to smell trouble. You believe in taking all necessary precautions to head it off.*

↑ Ⓣ *Tiwaz—The warrior goes bravely into battle. To hang on to the other things you value, you must be willing to fight to keep them. And so you value valor.*

↓ Ⓣ *Tiwaz reversed—The defeated warrior returns to fight another day. You value dignity and honor. You believe you can't keep a "good man" down. You'd like to meet Horatio Alger.*

U Ⓤ   **↑** Ⓝ   **B** Ⓑ

lUck   Need   Birth

2 To get ahead, you will need all the luck you can get . . . but get ahead you must—if not on your own, then with the help of your trio of Runes. The **U**-Rune provides you with an endless source of the good stuff—luck, that is. The **N**-Rune makes you want more and more. And the **B**-Rune sees you through the bad that yet may be turned to good—even if you brought some of your own woes upon yourself. In general, you appear to be a fairly lucky stiff. But your success actually comes from a combination of timely breaks and concerted efforts. You will amount to what you make the most of. Choose your values . . .

U Ⓤ *Uruz—The bull ox thrashes his way through the forest—and never mind the fences. You value your independence. You believe in your own Manifest Destiny.*

Π Ⓝ *Uruz reversed—The bull ox lowers his head, paws the earth, and snorts before he charges. You value a timely warning . . . and a friendly piece of advice. (Watch out for the Ⓔ Ⓢ !?) You believe in turf wars.*

✦ Ⓝ *Naudhiz—Need is always waiting below the surface like a persistent itch. And when it rises up, you value a good set of fingernails. You believe some lessons are only learned the hard way.*

Ƀ Ⓑ *Berkano—Birch trees, they say, bless the couple of the house with children. You value the birthing process itself, and every other act of creation. You believe in bringing your twinkling ideas to life.*

◣ Ⓖ *Berkano reversed—The young birches flail wildly in the wind, but they rarely snap. You value elasticity. And you believe it's possible to snap back from just about anything. You'd like to shake hands with the Hardy Boys.*

Þ ⓉⒽ   **I** Ⓘ   **M** Ⓔ

faiTh   Ice   fEmale

3 You can move mountains, my friend—and I kid you not. Your trinity of Runes is like a lever. The **Th**-Rune gives you all the faith you will ever need to do anything worthwhile. The **I**-Rune provides you with a will of steel that keeps you true to your word. And the **E**-Rune gives you the inspiration and trust you need to empower your prayers. You will amount to as much as you wish earnestly for. But you have a particular talent for self-improvement projects and public works. By sticking within certain limits and living within most of the rules, you will wind up accomplishing a goodly amount. You sure don't need anyone watching over your shoulder. Choose your values . . .

ᚦ Ⓣ *Thurisaz*—There are thorns so big, they warn you to stay back. You value those who keep a safe distance . . . or who can be seen coming. You believe in steering clear of the nails and veering past broken glass.

ᚦ Ⓣ *Thurisaz reversed*—There are thorns so small and insidious that they seem to reach out to get you. You value the opportunity to watch where you are going. You believe in proceeding with caution.

ᛁ Ⓘ *Isa*—The ice can be smooth and beautiful, but deceptively thin. You value the things that are tested and proven sure. You believe it's better to be safe than sorry. And you always ask for permission.

ᛗ Ⓔ *Ehwaz*—The mare gives birth to a colt in spring. You value each wholesome new beginning. You believe that the sun will rise tomorrow just as it always has before. And you believe in riding off into the sunset.

ᛠ Ⓔ *Ehwaz reversed*—The white stallion rears up on his hind legs. You value the pure, the pristine, and the additive-free. And you believe in saving wild things. You'd like to pet Bambi.

ᚠ Ⓐ   **◇** Ⓨ Ⓙ   **ᛗ** Ⓜ

fAte   Year   Male

4 Time is on your side, my friend . . . and you have a lifetime to use to your advantage. Your treble Runes provide the tools. The **A**-Rune gives you a good sense of who you are and what you can do. The **Y**-Rune provides you with the understanding of cause and effect. And the **M**-Rune gives you plenty of motivation. You learn from your experience and apply what you know. Given the time to pursue all your goals, you will surely achieve the most urgent ones. By the end, you will amount to whatever you have made of yourself during the sum total of your hours. Choose your values . . .

ᚠ Ⓐ *Ansuz*—The mouth gives words their shape, but it is the breath of life that gives them action. You value the power of the word to get things done. You believe in following the instructions.

ᚤ Ⓥ *Ansuz reversed*—The mouth has a mind of its own. You value the ability to change your mind sometimes. You believe in biting your tongue . . . and if not—well then—you can always take back your words.

ᚼ Ⓨ Ⓐ Ⓙ Ⓡ *Jera*—The year comes and goes, it seems, as fast as you can turn the pages in your book of days. You value the ability to plan your life in advance. You believe in schedules, calendars, and timetables.

ᛗ Ⓜ *Mannaz*—Human beings usually have a motive for the things they do and say. The question is, what's yours? You value your ability to reason. You believe in maintaining objectivity . . . even if it is subjective.

ᛉ Ⓦ *Mannaz reversed*—Human beings often say one thing and do something else. You value your lofty ideals. But you also believe in gray areas and judgment calls. You'd like to read Nixon's memoirs.

ᚱ Ⓡ　　　**ᛁ** Ⓔ　　　**ᛚ** Ⓛ

Reality　　　hElp　　　Love

5 Love heals all wounds, my friend . . . and erases old scars. And with this trident of Runes, you stand a good chance of coming out of it all hardly the worse for wear. The **R**-Rune lets you see things clearly—not only for what they are, but for what they could be. The Ê-Rune gives you the encouragement you need to stick with a project, through thick and thin. And the **L**-Rune gives you all the support you could ever care to muster to arms. You will amount to much, as long as the opinion of good friends and family members counts. In every respect, love creates its own reality. May you succeed in knowing yours. Choose your values . . .

R ® *Raidho*—The traveler sets out with nothing more than a few things in a bag. You value the time it takes to reach your destination. But you also value a scenic view.

◄ ⑼ *Raidho reversed*—The traveler returns with a head full of postcard pictures and a pair of widened eyes. You value the diversity of the life experience. But you also believe in buying round-trip tickets.

ϟ Ē Ɜ *Eihwaz*—The yew, they say, can live a thousand years. You value the things that are long-lived, time-tested, and centuries-proven. But you also believe in the miracles of modern science.

Γ Ⓛ *Laguz*—The high water flows among the trees and threatens the houses, but not the homes. You value that which goes on and on. You believe in keeping some things within the family.

◄ Ⓛ *Laguz reversed*—The low water opens up a passage to the far banks. You value the chance to expand into the new frontier. And you believe the grass is greener in Kentucky. You'd like to ride National Velvet.

◄ Ⓒ Ⓚ Ⓠ   **K** Ⓟ   **✖** Ⓝ

Course, Quest, Karma   hoPe   beING

6 Hope is the catalyst that eggs you on. So you are only encouraged by your triplicity of Runes. The **K**-Rune gives you a definite and specific sense of purpose. You know what you want. The **P**-Rune gives you the interest to step out on a limb and risk achieving it. And the **ING**-Rune gives you the creative energy to pursue the many dreams you are inclined to chase. It is by trial and error—and doing things until you get them right—that you achieve your purpose. You will amount to as much as you live and learn along the way. Choose your values . . .

◄ Ⓒ Ⓝ Ⓠ *Kenaz*—The Olympic torch burns with an eternal flame . . . but only for the length of the games. You value the things that symbolize your ideals. And you believe in keeping the home fires fueled.

> ⟩ Ⓖ Ⓨ Ⓞ *Kenaz reversed*—The fire that wavers may yet be saved. You value the things that, even if they flicker, still hint of the original flame. You believe in the saving of leftovers.

Ⓚ Ⓟ *Perthro*—When the dice are hot, it seems like they were never cold. You value the things that go out of their way to go yours. You believe it's possible to influence the outcome and stay on a roll.

Ⓚ Ⓓ *Perthro reversed*—When the dice are loaded, it doesn't matter how many times you say the magic words. You value a lesson learned on the street. You believe that life is a crapshoot.

Ⓧ Ⓝ *Ingwaz*—When the do-not-disturb sign is out, don't even think of knocking. You value the sanctity of your own boudoir. But you believe in pillow talk. You'd love to tune into Maury Povich.

Ⓧ Ⓖ   Ⓨ Ⓩ   Ⓡ Ⓞ

Gifts   reSIStance   hOme

7 You could not ask for more gifts than this triumvirate of Runes. The **G**-Rune gives you talents to discover, pursue, and exploit. The **Z**-Rune gives you the courage to keep at it all night. And the **O**-Rune supports you with a place to hang your hat. You will accomplish much of whatever you set out to do. You have many interests and outlets, and you receive much encouragement for your creative ideas. It's even possible that you will amount to more than you think. All you really need along the way is a little bit of timely luck to boost you on your way. Choose your values . . .

Ⓧ Ⓖ Ⓞ *Gebo*—A gift is a gift, regardless of price. You value the things that come in small boxes. But you also believe that some presents have too many strings attached.

Ⓨ Ⓩ *Elhaz*—The elk grows new antlers in the spring. You value the things that can come again when the winter is past. But you also believe some things are better held at bay.

Ⓐ Ⓩ *Elhaz reversed*—The elks butt antlers over a mate. You value the things that can come from a fight. And you believe that a handshake can make up for a lot of low blows.

⧓ Ⓞ *Othala—The house built on stilts withstands high tide. You value the things that are solid, time-honored, and dependable. You believe in keeping both feet planted squarely.*

⧓ Ⓞ *Othala reversed—A house built on fault lines may wind up on its roof. You value a firm floor beneath your bed. But you also believe that California is paradise. You'd like to swap places with Joe Hollywood.*

ᚠ Ⓥ Ⓦ   **ᛋ** Ⓢ   **ᛞ** Ⓓ

Wonder   Sun & Stars   Destiny

8 Just follow your bliss, my friend . . . that's all you need do. And with this trefoil of Runes behind you, you should have no problem blissing to your heart's content. The **W**-Rune gives you a love of life itself. The **S**-Rune gives you many bright things to marvel at. And the **D**-Rune allows you to find a purpose in even the common, the minor, and the mundane. You simply love the experience of being, doing, knowing, learning, seeing, sensing, feeling. Your destiny is woven up in the experience of achieving it. To say anything else right now would simply spoil the surprise. But yours will amount to a full life. Choose your values . . .

ᚠ Ⓥ Ⓦ *Wunjo—Life's best moments are the simplest, they say. You value life for the living it brings. But I can't tell whether you cook to live . . . or live to cook?[2] Believe what you will, my friend, it's your life span.*

◄ Ⓐ Ⓦ *Wunjo reversed—Life's little surprises are often ironic—yet you can't help but laugh. You value a little comic relief. And you believe it's important to look on the bright side.*

ᛋ Ⓢ *Sowilo—The sun goes and comes back again to mark each season in its turn. You value all the days of the year, but especially the holidays and weekends. You believe in both fasting and feasting.*

---

[2] . . . in the words of my Old Grandma—who at last count was 103. From her lips, it meant she'd rather read a book than fix dinner. But you can make of it as you please.

▶️◻️◻️ *Dagaz*—*The days tick off like an alarm clock. You value a good night's sleep. And you believe that things will look better in the morning. But you'd like to have a word with Father Time.*

◻️

weird

9 Wait and see, my friend, wait and see. The Blank Rune provides you with exponential possibilities. All the other Runes are here—upright and reversed—and every possible combination of them.[3] In a sense, you are a Jack of all trades . . . but a master of one. The hardest part for you is deciding what it is you want to do. What you amount to will depend on which decisions you make, and when. All ways, means, and ends are at your disposal. If in doubt, try out something new. Eventually you'll find what you're best at. The signs number just the one, but it is many . . .

◻️ *Weird*—*The Universe is a diverse and mysterious place . . . so is the world . . . and so are you. You value the unknown and unknowable. You believe that you were meant to do something with your life.*

EXTRA CREDIT

To get in touch with your morals. Gather your Runes together and mix them up while you think about the issue that you are confronting. Ask your question: **What do I value?** about my life in general? my mate? my job? **What morals are involved in my decision?** Or simply **Give me values.** Select the three Runes that come into your palm, or cast your Runes on the floor and pick three from the heap. Note whether they are upright or reversed, then look them up in this Reading's Answer section. Read the text in *italics*. Each Rune will give you a little something to think about with regard to your decision.

[3] If you select just two Runes at a time, there are 600 possible combinations. (They are all listed in Reading #9's Answer section.) Choose three Runes at once, and there are 13,800 possibilities. Four Runes at a time, 303,600 . . . five Runes, 6,375,600 . . . and my pocket calcualtor runs out of memory after that.

EXTRA, EXTRA CREDIT!

To play anagrams. Here's a fun diversion that will let your Runes speak directly to you. Simply gather all your Runes (or alphabet tiles) together and think of anything that's been on your mind. Say the magic words, **Spell it all out. Spell out what I should know about** _____. my love life. my home life. my work life. my secret life. Or simply say, **Speak to me.** Cast your Runes on the floor and jot down the letters of all those that land Rune side up. (Treat all reversed Runes as if they are upright). Then let the games begin.

Unscramble the letters you have received to see what words you can make of them. Use the letters as many times as needed. Then circle all the words in your list that click with you. Don't forget to look for people's names and initials. If your answer is unclear, draw one Rune at random and consult the Quick Reference Guide's Master Answer section.

Go on to the next Reading whenever you are ready to continue.

Reading #21

WHO DO I THINK I AM?
(Hocus-pocus, give me focus)

In this Reading, you'll add up the letters in your first name to get a glimpse of both your ego and your aura. You can also use this Reading to draw or cast Runes in order to keep your life in focus.

ᚠ ᚠ ᚠ

RUNE TOOLS

You don't need any new tools to do this Reading. But here's a cheat sheet to remind you of the Runes and their numerical values . . .

1	2	3	4	5	6	7	8
ᚠ	ᚢ	ᚦ	ᚨ	ᚱ	ᚲ	ᚷ	ᚠ
F	U	Th	A	R	C/K/Q	G	V/W
ᚺ	ᚾ	ᛁ	ᛃ	ᛇ	ᛈ	ᛉ	ᛊ
H	N	I	Y/J	Ê	P	Z	S
ᛏ	ᛒ	ᛖ	ᛗ	ᛚ	ᛜ	ᛟ	ᛞ
T	B	E	M	L	-ing	O	D

O = 9

HOW TO

To find out what the name you go by says about your self-image . . .

1   Go back to the Scratch Pad in Reading #6 and copy down the Runes for the name you go by. Or write your first name from scratch here.

Scratch Pad

Jot down your Runes here.

---

2   Now, for each and every Rune in your first name, jot down its corresponding number (1 through 9) from the chart in this Reading's Tools section.

Let's say your name is Mary Caroline, but you go by Mary. Translating Mary's name into Runes, it would look like this: ᛗᚠᚱᛢ. Since ᛗ (M) has a value of 4, Mary would jot down the number 4 under her M. Then, continuing: ᚠ (A) = 4, ᚱ (R) = 5, and ᛢ (Y) = 4.

3   Now add these numbers together. In Mary's case, 4 + 4 + 5 + 4 = 17. Keep adding until you've got a number between 1 and 9. For Mary, 1 + 7 = 8. Mary's number is 8. Look up your number in this Reading's Answer section.

As in Reading #20, your answer consists of three Runes, which the text will describe for you. The synopsis is followed by a list of "focal points." From among them, choose your focus for today.

THE ANSWERS

The Runes appear in their traditional numerical order, but they are list-ed in trios. Reversed Runes are listed under their upright counterparts (✕, ᚻ, ✝, ᛁ, ◇, ᛏ, ᛋ, ᛉ, ᛗ, and ☐ have no reversals).

F	U	Th	A	R	K	G	W
H	N	I	Y	Ê	P	Z	S
T	B	E	M	L	X	O	D	☐

K=C & Q; W=V; Y=J

ᚠ ᚢ ᚦ ᚨ ᚱ ᚲ ✕ ᚹ
ᚺ ✝ ᛁ ◇ ᛏ ᚲ ᚿ ᛋ
↑ ᛒ ᛗ ᛗ ᛚ ᛉ ᛟ ᛗ ☐

ᚠ Ⓕ   **ᚺ** Ⓗ   **↑** Ⓣ
Fortune   Hail   Triumph

1 **F, H,** and **T**—these three—give you an air of self-confidence. If you dress for success, others will automatically treat you with respect (at least to your face). If you speak in an authoritative voice, others will turn their heads (if only to glare). But package yourself as a force for good, and the floor is yours (at least for a day). You think of yourself as a go-getter, a get-things-doner, and maybe even a mover and shaker. Money and power go hand in hand—and you see nothing wrong with either of them. Together they give you the clout to feel important while you shop, eat, and attend to things. And if you're really lucky, others won't expect a big tip. Select your focus from these . . .

ᚠ Ⓕ *Fehu—The cattle are slow to move without a prod. When things refuse to go your way, try giving them a nudge. The focus is on getting things in motion. If you're done playing with your Runes, let's get start-ed.*

ᚠ Ⓕ *Fehu reversed—The cattle like to chew their cud. Find yourself something to keep your hands occupied and your mind busy. The focus is on staying active. Hup-one. Hup-two. Hup-three.*

N Ⓗ *Hail*—The storm needs to dump its load before it runs its course. Work off excess tension. Vent some frustration. Let off a little steam. The focus is on achieving equilibrium.

↑ Ⓣ *Tiwaz*—The soldier needs discipline as well as nerve, but mostly it's a matter of quick reflexes. Respond to each and every threat. React to each new volley. The focus is on thinking fast . . . and acting quicker.

↓ Ⓣ *Tiwaz reversed*—The soldier needs some R and R from active duty. Take a load off. Put your feet up. The focus is on calculated inaction. Hold hands with your remote.

U Ⓤ   **↑** Ⓝ   **B** Ⓑ

lUck   Need   Birth

2 U, N, and **B**—these three—give you an aura of determination. If you watch out for miracles, you will see them all the time. If you watch for mysteries, there are still plenty to unravel. And if you look for demons, you will find them, too. You think of yourself as a lucky person (knock on wood). And in many respects you are charmed. But it is mostly by your cunning that you get by. If you are really lucky, you'll be able to get away with murder (but if I were you, I wouldn't try). Select your focus for today from these . . .

U Ⓤ *Uruz*—The bull ox lets nothing get in his way . . . at least not for long. Adopt a winning stance. Assume the position. Crack down. The focus is on breaking your way clean through these human barriers.

∩ Ⓝ *Uruz reversed*—The bull ox puts on a roaring good show. When there is no room for negotiation, bluff or be bluffed. The focus is on maneuvering. If all else fails, play politics.

↑ Ⓝ *Naudhiz*—Need causes folks to do things they otherwise wouldn't. Think twice before doing what you otherwise shouldn't. The focus is on coming through it all in one piece. Do what you gotta.

ᛒ ⓑ *Berkano*—The birches stand out white against the dark backdrop of the forest. Hold up your head. Stand tall. And rise above the rest. The focus is on growth. Develop height, girth, and depth.

ᛒ ⑨ *Berkano reversed*—The birch switch stings the contrite flesh. When need be, take your punishment. Ask for forgiveness. The focus is on wiping the slate clean. Take this chance to start all over again.

ᚦ ⓣʰ   **ᛁ** ⓘ   **ᛗ** ⓔ

faiTh   Ice   fEmale

3 Th, I, and E—these three—make you seem like a person who has plenty of muscle. If you walk the line, others will tug you along with them. If you slip too near the line, others will pull you back. But if you cross over the line, others will be inclined to leave you flat. You think of yourself as a team player. And so you are guided by the rules. Not that they are easy, mind you, or that you don't commit a foul once in a while. But under these conditions, it is by feet and inches that progress is made, and not by leaping bounds. If you are really lucky, the opposition will be weak. Select your focus for today from these . . .

ᚦ ⓣʰ *Thurisaz*—The thorn has no compunction about going for blood. Sometimes you, too, have to be pricked to wake up. The focus is on protecting your own interests. Trust your better judgment.

ᚦ ⓣʰ *Thurisaz reversed*—The barb hangs on and won't let loose. The focus is on getting out from under something that holds you down, back, or fast. Remove the thorn from your own side first. Then untangle the larger mess.

ᛁ ⓘ *Isa*—The ice is so cold, it burns the flesh as effectively as fire, but leaves less-lasting marks. The focus is on getting beneath the surface. If nothing else works, try psychology. Learn how to push the cold as well as the hot buttons.

M Ⓔ *Ehwaz*—The horse works up quite a sweat. If you must perspire, don't let 'em see you. The focus is on keeping a cool head. Champ at the bit if you must, but harness your resources. One, two, three, pull.

W Ⓔ *Ehwaz reversed*—The horse loses a shoe. Hang it over your doorway, for goodness' sake. The focus is on staying out of trouble. Keep your hands to yourself. Mind your own business. Keep your stable clean.

ᚠ Ⓐ   **ᛃ** Ⓨ Ⓙ   **ᛗ** Ⓜ

fAte   Year   Male

4 A, Y, and M—these three—give you the look of a proud and accomplished person. If you wish to be the captain of your fate, you must learn to navigate first. If you wish to be the reaper of your just reward, you first must plant. But if you wish to be the master of your soul, you need only take the reins. Whether you think of yourself as an under- or an overachiever, a results-oriented kind, or an unfortunate one, it shows on the surface. And nine times out of ten it is a self-fulfilling prophecy. If you are really lucky, you will get to have all three of your wishes come true. Select your focus for today from these . . .

ᚠ Ⓐ *Ansuz*—In the beginning was the word . . . and it was "go." So on your marks, get ready . . . get set. The focus is on the power of the word to set things in motion. Just say it.

ᚨ Ⓥ *Ansuz reversed*—In the end was the word . . . and it too was "go." All systems are set for reentry sequence. Okay. Roger. And out. The focus is on getting in the last word. What is it?

ᛃ Ⓨ Ⓐ Ⓙ Ⓘ *Jera*—Solstice to solstice and equinox to equinox, the four seasons come, go, and come back around . . . and around. Set some benchmarks. The focus is on getting the timing down right.

ᛗ Ⓜ *Mannaz*—The man who gets the job done has put in a fair day's labor for his pay. The focus is on getting what you deserve. And fair's fair. Earn your own way, have your own say.

ᛗ Ⓦ *Mannaz reversed*—The man who sleeps on the job gets paid any-way. They also serve who only supervise. The focus is on minding your own business. Don't worry about what somebody else is getting away with.

ᚱ Ⓡ   **ᛇ Ⓔ**   **ᛚ Ⓛ**

Reality   hElp   Love

5 R, Ê, and L—these three—give you the air of someone who is sincere, honest, loyal, and earnestly trying to do the right thing. If you go off looking for the truth, you will more than likely find your own version of it. If you ask others for their opinion, they will glad-ly give their two cents worth (which is about its street value). But if you would really find your true love, you must let it find you. You think of yourself as someone who has a higher purpose. And we all do. But with these Runes behind your name, you are sure to latch on to yours. If you're really lucky, others will think it's important too. Choose your focus for today from these . . .

ᚱ Ⓡ *Raidho*—The road goes on forever, with two lanes in either direc-tion and a median strip up the center. You need to watch for your exit. The focus is on speed limits and mile markers. Pass only with care.

ᚱ Ⓦ *Raidho reversed*—The road comes abruptly to a dead end. When you get lost, retrace your steps. The focus is on following directions. Look for familiar landmarks. Feel your way back on course.

ᛇ Ⓔ *Eihwaz*—The yew does not lose its leaves nor change its color. And thrown upon the fire, it sputters. Feel for the spark within you. The focus is on being true to yourself. Only then can you work your magic.

ᛚ Ⓛ *Laguz*—The springwater that drips from the rock face into the bottles is pure and clear. Keep yourself clean, inside and out. The focus is on personal hygiene. Purify yourself before you make overtures.

↙ ⌐ *Laguz reversed*—The liquid is brackish that comes from the tap. *Travel near and far, but don't drink the water. The focus is on preventive measures. Before you operate, sterilize the utensils.*

< ⌐ Ⓚ Ⓠ   Ⱪ Ⓟ   ✗ Ⓧ

Course, Quest, **Katma**   hoPe   beING

6 C, **P**, and **-ing**—these three—give you the aura of someone who is rather naïve. If you think of the world as a place where truth and light win out, you'll find an example or two of a good guy who didn't finish last. If you think, for all its sham and drudgery, it's still a beautiful place, you'll catch sight of an occasional rainbow. But if you think it's all about romance, you may be in for a rude awakening. You think of yourself as a person who can see the good in everyone and everything. But you might have to remove a few top layers first. If you're really lucky, you won't be disappointed when you get down to the core. Choose your focus for today from these . . .

< ⌐ Ⓚ Ⓠ *Kenaz*—*The sunlight is so bright, it warms even the nooks and crannies of the house. When you go out looking for the truth, better bring along your dark glasses. The focus is on finding things out for yourself. Be ready for an education as well as an enlightenment.*

> ⌐ Ⓚ Ⓠ *Kenaz reversed*—*The moonlight is so bright, you could read a book by it. But take it easy on yourself . . . you wouldn't want to go blind. The focus is on keeping it all within reasonable limits . . . especially in the dark.*

Ⱪ Ⓟ *Perthro*—*The dice come up 7's and 11's. You win! Take the opportunity to cash in your chips. The focus is on playing things close to your vest and quitting while you're still ahead.*

↘ ⌐ *Perthro reversed*—*The dice come up snake eyes. You lose! Care to double your wager? The focus is on winning things back. But remember, two times zero is less than one.*

✗ Ⓧ *Ingwaz*—*Someone's got to come out on top. Take your time. Don't jump the gun. And never cheat on a good thing. The focus is on erogenous zones. (What's that unsightly mark on your neck?)*

✗ Ⓖ   ᛉ Ⓩ   ᛟ Ⓞ

Gifts   reSIStance   hOme

7 G, Z, and O—these three—give you an aura of human decency. If you play nice and share your toys with others, things will go better for all parties concerned. If you stick up for your buddies, you can hold off the bullies. And if you help out around the house, you may even get an allowance. You think of yourself as one of the "good guys." And with a name like this, you deserve a white hat. You may not wind up with much else, but at least it will be a quality life. And if you're really lucky, others will treat you as well as you treat them. Select your focus for today from these . . .

✗ Ⓖ Ⓖ *Gebo—A gift is like a favor that needs to be repaid. Honor your commitments. Pay your debts. And when in doubt, buy presents. The focus is on coming out even, if not ahead. Be fair. Be square. Obey the laws of the pack.*

ᛉ Ⓩ *Elhaz—The elk seeks the company of others only when it's time to mate. You, too, must fight—or be fought over—for the privilege. The focus is on passing the initiation. There is something you need to prove to others—or is it to yourself?*

ᛦ Ⓩ *Elhaz reversed—The elk travels alone most of the time. You, too, could stand a stint at living off the land. The focus is on gathering up your inner strength and moral courage. Retreat into yourself. Mend. Heal. Replenish.*

ᛟ Ⓞ *Othala—Home is the place where everybody knows the name you go by. So choose the name that fits you . . . and suits your purpose. The focus is on family, friends, and everyone who loves you just the way you are.*

ᛟ Ⓞ *Othala reversed—Home is the place you'd really rather be. So make time to be there. And make time to get out and do something as a family for a change. The focus is on keeping your own house in order.*

ᚠ ⟨ᚡ⟩ ᚹ   ᛋ ⟨ᛋ⟩   ᛗ ⟨ᛞ⟩

Wonder   Sun & Stars   Destiny

---

8 W, S, and D—these three—give you the air of a person who makes the most out of life. If you take a break once in a while, you will see that there is more than working nine to six. If you look up at the sky now and again, you will be reminded of what lasts. And if you take each day as it comes, you will make it through most of them. I guarantee it. You may think of yourself as the easygoing, fun-loving type. And why not get your kicks? But if you're going to take a deep breath, remember to exhale. If you're really lucky, others will laugh with you. Choose your focus for today from these . . .

ᚠ ⟨ᚡ⟩ ᚹ *Wunjo—Joy cometh in the morning.[1] Be up and doing in the dawn's early light. Get out and about. The focus is on being the first in line. Whistle while you work.*

◁ ⟨ᚠ⟩ ᚹ *Wunjo reversed—Weeping doth not last the night. Dream your cares away, call in sick, and sleep in late. The focus is on getting better. Guard your mental health. Come back to life.*

ᛋ ⟨ᛋ⟩ *Sowilo—Who can loose the bands of Orion?[2] Learn to live with the things that only God can change. Despite what ails or annoys you, the days arrive and go away. The focus is on seeing past the distractions.*

ᛗ ⟨ᛞ⟩ ⟨ᛋ⟩ *Dagaz—Day unto day . . . and night unto night.[3] Ashes to ashes . . . and dust to dust. Learn what you can and experience the rest. The focus is on going home at the end of the day . . . older, richer, and wiser for the wear.*

[1] Psalms 23:5
[2] Job 28:31
[3] Psalms 19:2

◻

weird

9 The Blank Rune gives you an air of mystery, an aura of mystique, and a certain enchanting quality. If you see it all as an endless set of possibilities for things to go right, you will never lack for motivation. If you see it all as a string of reasons why things could go wrong, you will never want for excuses. And if you see both pro and con in everything, you will never finish your list. No one is more charming than you. But you also have a flaky quality. If you're really lucky, people will give you credit for just showing up and giving it your best shot. Your winning formula is tried but true . . .

◻ *Weird—So you're not like everybody else. Around here it's okay to be different. The focus is on self-expression. Keep to yourself if you like. Be eccentric if you want. Find like-minded friends.*

EXTRA CREDIT

To set your sights. Gather your Runes together while you think about the challenges and opportunities that confront you. Say, **Hocus-pocus, give me focus.** Or, **Give me some focus about _____.** Select three Runes all at once. Line them up in front of you and check to see whether each is upright or reversed. Look them up in this Reading's Answer section. Consult the *italic* portion of the text. The three Runes together will tell you three things you need to focus on.

EXTRA, EXTRA CREDIT!

Looking for a mate? a job? a raise? Mix up all your Runes while you think of the goal you want to achieve. Say, **Pretty please, give me some leads.** Then select the three Runes that feel right and place them faceup in front of you. Look up your Runes in the Master Answer section at the back of the book and read the Love, Work, or Money section of the text, as appropriate. The Strategy section will also add to your understanding of any answer.

Go on to the next Reading whenever you are ready to continue.

Reading #22

WHAT'S MY INNER MAGIC?
(Guide my footsteps)

In this Reading, you will add up the Runes of your middle name to
learn about your secrets to success. Or you can use this Reading to
draw or cast Runes in order to resolve a current difficulty,
step by step.

✸ ✸ ✸

RUNE TOOLS

Here's a handy chart that summarizes the Futhark's three tiers (reading left to right) of eight Runes each . . .

	1	2	3	4	5	6	7	8
1	F	U	Th	A	R	C/K/Q	G	V/W
2	H	N	I	Y/J	Ê	P	Z	S
3	T	B	E	M	L	-ing	O	D

□ = 9

. . . as well as the corresponding Rune trios they form, reading top to
bottom. In this Reading, we'll be making use of the trios again.

HOW TO

To learn about your inner magic, just . . .

1 Turn back to Reading #7, where you wrote your middle name in Runes, and copy it down here. Or write your middle name in Runes from scratch . . .

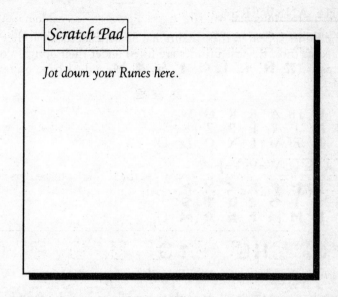

Scratch Pad

Jot down your Runes here.

2 Now look up each of your Runes in the table in this Reading's Tools section. Find its number value (1 through 8) along the top of the chart. And jot it down on the scratch pad.

Richard's middle name is (shh! don't tell anyone) Isaiah. So Richard Isaiah would convert his "secret" name to Runes and numbers like this: I/ **I** = <u>3</u>; S/**ϟ** = <u>8</u>; A/**ᚨ** = <u>4</u>; I/ **I** = <u>3</u>; A/**ᚨ** = <u>4</u>; H/**ᚺ** = <u>1</u>.

3 Once you've copied down all your numbers, add them up to get a total. The total will probably be a two-digit number. Now add one digit to the other to get a final number between 1 and 9.

In Richard Isaiah's case: 3 + 8 + 4 + 3 + 4 + 1 = 23. Then, reducing the total: 2 + 3 = 5. Richard Isaiah's number is 5. He'd look it up in this Reading's Answer section. Now's a good time to look up yours.

As in Readings #20 and #21, your answer will include three Runes. Read the main text, which describes your three Runes in combination. Then select your secret weapon for today from the list of tools that follows.

THE ANSWERS

The Runes appear in their traditional numerical order, but they are listed in trios. Reversed Runes are listed under their upright counterparts (✕, ᚺ, ✛, ᛁ, ◇, ↑, ᛋ, ✳, ᛗ, and ⬡ have no reversals).

F	U	Th	A	R	K	G	W
H	N	I	Y	Ê	P	Z	S
T	B	E	M	L	X	O	D	⬡

K=C & Q; W=V; Y=J

ᚠ ᚢ ᚦ ᚨ ᚱ ᚲ ᚷ ᚹ
ᚺ ᚾ ᛁ ◇ ↑ ᛉ ᛃ ᛋ
↑ ᛒ ᛗ ᛘ ᛚ ᛜ ᛟ ᛞ ⬡

ᚠ Ⓕ   ᚺ Ⓗ   ↑ Ⓣ

Fortune   Hail   Triumph

1 It has something to do with the spoils of war, my friend. The things you would possess will come to you only after a fight . . . and only if you win. Your secrets to success are three: You have the power to go after anything you desire. You have the power to use force if need be. And you have the power to come out on top, smelling like a rose. It is your underlying aggressive nature that gets you into trouble . . . as well as out. Mind your temper. Watch your words. Look over your shoulder. Don't take anything or anyone for granted. Be on guard. Choose your secret weapon . . .

ᚠ Ⓕ *Fehu—The cattle are collateral. To get by, you too will need assets—if only a few. The things that you already possess are your best weapons. Make your money work for you. Invest it wisely.*

◢ Ⓕ *Fehu reversed*—The cattle are chattel. Sell off the things you no longer need. Turn liquid assets into greenbacks. Your secret weapon is cash on the hoof . . . on hand . . . and in reserve.

H Ⓗ *Hail*—The hail does its work quickly and professionally. In a sudden outburst, you too can wreak much havoc in only a few words. Your secret weapon is a well-aimed barb. Leave no blood.

↑ Ⓣ *Tiwaz*—The fighter returns a hero from the war. In a crisis you too are capable of rising to the fore. Your secret weapons are fist, foot, tooth, and nail. But with your brains you will prevail.

↓ Ⓣ *Tiwaz reversed*—The soldier tries to go down fighting—if go down, he must. You too may falter or fail in your gallant attempts. Your secret weapon is a white flag. If worst comes to worst, wave it thrice o'er your pretty head.

Ʋ Ⓤ   ✝ Ⓝ   ᛒ Ⓑ

lUck   Need   Birth

2 It has something to do with the odds being what they are, my friend. What you would make of yourself all depends on what opportunities knock. Your secrets to success are these: You have the power to take advantage of a winning streak. You have the power to ride out a losing streak. And, if all else fails, you have the power to try, try again. It is your winning spirit that prevails in the end. Take what comes. Play along with the game. Do the best that you can. Choose your secret weapon . . .

Ʋ Ⓤ *Uruz*—The bull ox has a great pair of horns. And lucky for you they are pointed up. Tempt not the fates nor court disaster. Your secret weapon is a lucky hat . . . and your own thick skull. Stay lucky.

∩ Ⓤ *Uruz reversed*—The bull ox—how should I put it?—is well endowed. If you've got it, flaunt it, I guess. Your secret weapon is in your pants. But don't let it do <u>all</u> your thinking for you. Get lucky.

✦ Ⓝ *Naudhiz*—The need is great. You must rise above it all . . . or else transcend. Your secret weapon is a vivid imagination. Paint pictures. Dream dreams. Imagine you are someplace else. Escape into a fantasy.

ᛒ Ⓑ *Berkano*—The birches are the first to green in spring. You too are fertile, fecund, and prolific. Your secret weapon is the urge itself. Let your creative juices stir—or is it stew? Give birth to an idea.

ᛊ Ⓖ *Berkano reversed*—The birch loses its bark to blight, but yet endures. You too are capable of pulling through. Your secret weapon is adaptability. Blend in. Adopt a new name. Assume a new identity.

ᚦ Ⓣⱨ   **ᛁ Ⓘ**   **ᛗ Ⓔ**
faiTh   Ice   fEmale

3 It has as much to do with the forces outside you as within you. The things you want to do—or not do—come as a result of your own actions and counteractions. You have three secrets to success: You have the ability to call on powers greater than yourself. You have the ability to block out negative influences. And you have the ability to listen to your own conscience. It is your beliefs that see you through. Trust in your God. Pray. Call. Summon. Invoke. Resist those who would interfere with your religious freedom. Listen to your spirit guides. Choose your secret weapon . . .

ᚦ Ⓣⱨ *Thurisaz*—Life is no bed of roses . . . unless you don't mind sleeping with thorns. It all depends on what position you take. Your secret weapon is belief. What you see is what you get.

ᚦ Ⓣⱨ *Thurisaz reversed*—It's like walking on glass or sleeping on a bed of nails. It's 99% mind over matter, you know. You secret weapon is faith. Meet a challenge. Pass a test. Practice what you preach.

ᛁ Ⓘ *Isa*—The ice is black as blood in the moonlight. Take care and use all necessary caution. Your secret weapon is a healthy respect, which some might call fear. But here's your chance to walk on water.

M Ⓔ *Ehwaz*—*The horse gives warning of a coming storm. You too can feel the weather changing in your bones. Your secret weapon is in knowing a sign when you see it. Ask for a hint. Look for the message.*

W Ⓔ *Ehwaz reversed*—*The horse will not go willingly through a burning barn. Never doubt your own instincts. Your secret weapon is common sense. Listen to the voice of reason in your head.*

ᚠ Ⓐ   **◇** Ⓨ Ⓙ   **ᛗ** Ⓜ

fAte   Year   Male

4 It has as much to do with words as deeds. The things you want to achieve in your lifetime come as a result of thoughts as well as actions. Your secrets to success are three: You have the power to speak your mind and make your desires known. You have the power to observe how things typically happen. And you have the power to learn how things get accomplished. It is your ability to read, write, and cipher that gets the job done. Speak distinctly and clearly—but only raise your voice if they can't hear you from the back of the room. Follow the instructions in the book. Do first things first. And clean up when you're done. Choose your secret weapon . . .

ᚠ Ⓐ *Ansuz*—*The poem says it all in a few words. You too are able to get your point across succinctly. Your secret weapon is not the sword but the pen. Organize your thoughts. Package your message.*

ᚠ Ⓜ *Ansuz reversed*—*The words overflow from the computer. As long as you can scan, you're set. Your secret weapon is a highlighter. Find the main points. Jump to the summary. Reach a conclusion.*

◇ Ⓨ Ⓐ Ⓙ Ⓕ *Jera*—*Where one year lets off, a new year starts. Do a little at a time and you will get done by the deadline. Your secret weapon is the time that's on your side. Make the most of each and every day and night.*

ᛗ Ⓜ *Mannaz—Human beings are capable of much. Take the wisdom of your race and apply it. Your secret weapon is a lesson from history. Build on the trials and errors of the past. Add to the record books.*

ᛝ Ⓦ *Mannaz reversed—Human beings are mere mortals. Don't take anyone or anything for granted. Your secret weapon is the will to survive. Much can be done in a single lifetime. But go for it now.*

ᚱ Ⓡ   ᛇ Ⓔ   ᛚ Ⓛ

Reality   **hElp**   **Love**

5 It has something to do with not giving up easily. The things you want to discover are mostly about yourself. Your secret to success involves three things: You have the power to search out the answers for yourself. You have the power to stand on your own two feet and defend yourself. And you have the power to connect to sources outside yourself. It is your mission that keeps you plugging. Be realistic, but not to a fault. Leave room for optimism, ideals, and things of the heart. Go when you must. Return when you can. And drive safely both ways. Choose your secret weapon . . .

ᚱ Ⓡ *Raidho—The traveler carries a good-luck piece. You too would do well to wear protection. Your secret weapon is your personal charm. Use your craft, skill, wit, and wisdom. Find things that are lost.*

ᚴ Ⓨ *Raidho reversed—The traveler is detoured, diverted, or otherwise delayed. Learn to make use of unscheduled downtime. Your secret weapon is a pair of thumbs. Employ your idle hands. Direct your idle mind.*

ᛇ Ⓔ Ⓔ *Eihwaz—The bow made of yew is strong yet resilient. When you get bent out of shape, snap back. Your secret weapon is inner strength. Connect to the source of your inspiration. Hit your mark.*

ᛚ Ⓛ *Laguz—The tide comes and goes with the moon. Watch, too, for the tides to rise and fall in you. Your secret weapon is in the power of your dreams. Employ your subconscious. Let it do its work for you.*

↓⌐ *Laguz reversed*—The open sea is unpredictable. Be wary of the creatures that lurk in the deep . . . and the waves that form from out of nowhere. Your secret weapon is to hold on for dear life. Stick to an even keel.

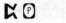

Course, Quest, Karma   hoPe   beING

6 It has something to do with all the pieces falling into place. The things you want to know have a way of revealing themselves in enlightening ways. Your secrets to success are these: You have the power to know the truth when you see it. You have the power to find guidance from the Runes. You have the power to act on your instincts, hunches, and intuition. But it is your vision that sees you through. Be open and receptive. Take a calculated risk or two. Direct your energies. Channel your sexual urge. Choose your secret weapon . . .

< © Ⓝ Ⓠ *Kenaz*—The light dispels the darkness. The day displaces night. Do what you will, but head for the light. Your secret weapon is a built-in homing device. Go on automatic pilot. Switch to cruise control.

> Ⓞ Ⓝ Ⓢ *Kenaz reversed*—The light fades. Look into your heart for the answer, and ken it well. Your secret weapon is the ability to read between the lines. Make inferences. Reach conclusions on your own.

Ⓚ Ⓟ *Perthro*—The dice cup is made from a fruit-bearing tree. For best results, so are the Runes. Your secret weapon is beginner's luck. Reach into the hat. Choose the numbers of your fate. Pick a winner.

Ⓧ Ⓓ *Perthro reversed*—The dice cup is turned out. And the Runes from your own hand spill to the floor. Your secret weapon is the ability to pick things out. Weave a story out of whole cloth. Stumble on the truth.

⊠ Ⓧ *Ingwaz—The earth is fertile . . . and all that dwell therein. You too are meant to be fruitful and multiply. Your secret weapon is in the seed of an idea. Plant yours. Care for your own. Work miracles.*

✕ Ⓖ   **Ψ Ⓩ**   **⊠ Ⓞ**

Gifts   reSIStance   hOme

7 It has something to do with networking. The security that you seek comes as a result of working with and through others. Your secrets to success are these: You have the power to combine resources to get the job done. You have the power to ward off danger by achieving safety in numbers. And together you have the power to erect a shelter from the cold and damp. It is your cooperative spirit that gets you what you want. Give and take. Do what's fair. Keep your honor. Chip in. Pay tribute. Choose your secret weapon . . .

✕ Ⓖ Ⓞ *Gebo—A gift is a small sacrifice to make. Be generous with the things you own, the thoughts you send, and the sentiments you feel. Your secret weapon is a present. Give it freely, openly, and without regret.*

Ψ Ⓩ *Elhaz—The elk uses its antlers as a defense. To ward off evil, splay your fingers and hold it back with the palm of your hand. Your secret weapon is the word "halt." Learn where to draw the line. Speak with conviction.*

⋏ Ⓩ *Elhaz reversed—The elk can still fight without its antlers. You too may need to paw, kick, spit, and scrape. Your secret weapon is surprise. Turn the other cheek if you can. But if need be, hit 'em where it hurts.*

⊠ Ⓞ *Othala—The house sits best in a clearing. Mark your boundaries and stake your claim to the surroundings. Your secret weapon is good fences. Establish limits. Color in the lines. Play within bounds.*

❖ ᛟ *Othala reversed*—The house is hidden from view. There is safety in obscurity. Your secret weapon is a low profile. Keep your secrets to yourself. Guard a family recipe. Keep your skeletons in the closet.

ᚠ ᚢ ᚹ   ᛋ   ᛞ

Wonder   Sun & Stars   Destiny

8 It is mostly a matter of seeing and believing. The things you want out of life are no different from the things your life already offers. You have three secrets to success: You have the power to enjoy your world as it is. You have the power to take each new day as it comes. And you have the power to go along for the ride. It is your trust in a higher purpose that gets you by. Take your time. Use your eyes, ears, nose, and lips. See. Taste. Touch. And feel. Take it all in. Treasure the moments, and remember them always. Choose your secret weapon . . .

ᚠ ᚢ ᚹ *Wunjo*—Glory comes to those who are willing to sacrifice. You too must put your life on the line in order to live it. Your secret weapon is strength in reserve. He who laughs lots, lives best.

◀ ᚢ ᚹ *Wunjo reversed*—Happiness comes to those who are willing to wait. But while you're busy waiting, don't forget that each day is a beauty. Your secret weapon is a wish. Close your eyes. And blow the dandelion seeds.

ᛋ *Sowilo*—Sun is the destroyer of ice, the drier of rain, and the tanner of flesh. Observe the powers of nature. Meld with your environment. Your secret weapon is plenty of fresh air. Breathe deep.

ᛞ *Dagaz*—The new day begins at midnight. Turn off the lights. Put out the cat. And snuggle in. Your secret weapon is a good long rest. Be early to bed and early to rise. Or else sleep in, and stay up late.

◻

weird

9 It has something to do with being open-minded. Though you are not always exactly sure of what it is you want, you are willing to consider the possibilities. The secret to your success is three-fold: You have the power to try out new things as they come. You have the power to choose your own cup of tea. You have the power to become just about anything that suits you. It is your willingness to try that makes it all possible. Give things the time they need to materialize. Build on the past. Live in the present. Create your own future. Your secret weapon is . . .

◻ *Weird—Things work in mysterious ways. Tap into the source. Pull down the energy. Put it to the task. Perform wonders. Work miracles. Believe in magic. Do the impossible . . . as if it were easy.*

EXTRA CREDIT

To identify the tools you need. Mix up your Runes while you think of the matter or issue that concerns you most right now. Ask the question **What tools do I need to do this deed?** Reach into your Runes and select as many as you like—two or three should do the trick. Then line them up in front of you. Together they comprise your Runic arsenal of "secret weapons." Look up each in this Reading's Answer section. Read the *italic* portion of the text. For good measure carry these Runes around in your pocket or purse for a day or two. And good luck to you.

EXTRA, EXTRA CREDIT!

To get out of a pickle. Mix up all your Runes while you think of the problem that you face (work, home, love, money, or whatever). Say the magic words: **Guide my footsteps.** Then draw the first three Runes that come into your hand. Place them in front of you in a line.

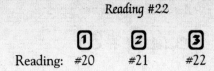

Reading: #20   #21   #22

Look up your Runes, as indicated, in Readings #20, #21, and #22. Read the *italic* portion of the text for your Rune, upright or reversed. Together the three will size up your situation and tell you what to do.

Go on to the next Reading whenever you are ready to continue.

Reading #23

WHAT'S MY LOT IN LIFE?
(Que sera sera)

In this Reading, you will add up <u>all</u> the letters in <u>all</u> your names to find the single Rune that is your mascot in life. You can also use this Reading to draw or cast Runes in order to determine the fate of just about anything.

ᛤ ᛤ ᛤ

RUNE TOOLS

Since the Blank Rune is a 20th-century invention, it has no standard place in the ancient Futhark sequence. We've been using it as the 25th Rune. But you could also think of it as the 1st Rune. You could place in the middle of the sequence. Or you could even think of it as being in position "0." This Reading's Answer section performs a little Rune-ological trick, by using the Blank Rune in all four places at once . . .

0	▢	7	ᚲ	14	▢	21	ᛗ
1	▢	8	ᚷ	15	ᛈ	22	ᛉ
2	ᚠ	9	ᚹ	16	ᛇ	23	ᛚ
3	ᚢ	10	ᚺ	17	ᛦ	24	ᛝ
4	ᚦ	11	ᚾ	18	ᛋ	25	ᛤ
5	ᚨ	12	ᛁ	19	ᛏ	26	ᛞ
6	ᚱ	13	ᛃ	20	ᛒ	27	▢

308

HOW TO

To find out which single Rune your whole name adds up to . . .

1 Go back to the Scratch Pads in Readings #20, #21, and #22 and copy down the numbers (1 through 9) you got when you added up your family name (Reading #20), the first name you go by (Reading #21), and your middle name (Reading #22). Jot these totals down on this Reading's Scratch Pad and you're ready to begin.

Scratch Pad

Jot down your numbers here.

---

2 Now, just add your three numbers together. Your total will be a number between 1 and 27.

3 Look up your number in this Reading's Answer section and find your lot in life. You can also consult the Quick Reference Guide's Master Answer section for more information about your Rune. In fact, you can look up your Rune in any Reading in this book, if you like. All the answers for your Rune pertain in some way to you.

THE ANSWERS

The answers appear—more or less—in the traditional order of the Runes, with additional Blank Runes added at the beginning and in the middle. Look up your answer by the number.

▢	F	U	Th	A	R	K	G	W	H	N	I	Y
▢	Ê	P	Z	S	T	B	E	M	L	X	O	D	▢

K=C & Q; W=V; Y=J

weirdest of the weird

0 You are not only **WEIRD**, but I can see you're the life of the party, Charlie. The only way you could have gotten this answer is if you did your math wrong. Or else it must be that you have no name whatsoever that you want to go by here. Why is it you choose to remain anonymous? Or do you have amnesia? Your lot, my friend, is: Sleep it off.

very weird

1 You are **WEIRD**, the extraordinary one. And I can see that you are one in a billion, all right. But why do you go by only the one name, Madonna?[1] And is it your first, middle, or last? You must either be very recognizable or awfully famous. How is it that you are able to command such popularity? And how does it feel to have all eyes focused on you? Your lot, my friend, is: A mystery to me.

Fortune.

2 You are **FEHU**, the one with many possessions . . . and so powerful, it seems, that you need only two names—or is it two initials,

[1] If this is not the case, OOPS! You have added incorrectly. Check out the How To section again.

J.R.?— for people to know who you are.[2] I see you will be a collector. But what is your collection? And how much is it worth? Certainly something is priceless to you. But what might that be? This, my friend, is thy lot: To find the one who will make your name—and life—complete.

ᚢ Ⓤ

lUck

3 You are **URUZ**, the free-spirited one . . . So, I see, it's difficult to hold you back or tie you down. Why do I see you changing residences—again and again? Do you go as the spirit leads you? As the fates befall? Or as luck would have it? And what do you do once you get there? Do you think maybe somebody is trying to tell you something? This, my friend, is thy lot: To lead the Gypsy life.

ᚦ Ⓣⱨ

faiTh

4 You are **THURISAZ**, the pious one. And yes, I see you down on bended knee and praying earnestly. But what? Is this the Crystal Cathedral? Through the glass I thought I saw trees. Oh well, the question is: What keeps you coming back? Your sin? Or your sanity? Do the answers elude you . . . or just the questions? What's it say in the book? Your lot, my friend, is: The path of the Pilgrim.

ᚠ Ⓐ

fAte

5 You are **ANSUZ**, the one of words. That's probably why I see you with an open book in your lap. But why are you writing with a feather? Do you take pride in penmanship? Or do you just like calligraphy? And what's that song that you can't get out of your head? Does the word touch you so much? And can't it make you laugh as well as cry? Your lot, my friend, is: The soul of a poet.

---

[2] The only way to get a "2" is if you're only using two names and they each add up to "1." Redo your math if it's not true of you.

ᚱ Ⓡ

Reality

6 You are **RAIDHO**, the one that journeys. And the way you choose is your own. I see you going by land, by sea, and even sky. But why are you alone? Could it be that there is something left for you to prove? Hear? Witness? See? Is it all out there? Or is it all in you? What do your little voices tell you? Your lot, my friend, is: To return from the wilderness.

ᚲ Ⓒ Ⓚ Ⓠ

Course, Quest, Karma

7 You are **KENAZ**, the one of deeds. And I see clearly now, it is as much what you do as what you did. You are turning the prayer wheel. But what is your penance? Or else, what favor do you ask? And are you motives pure? Your thoughts sincere? Who were you in a former life? And what are you coming back as? Your lot, my friend, is: Exactly what you asked for.

ᚷ Ⓖ

Gifts

8 You are **GEBO**, the gifted one. And I see you reading the signs into everything. I even see you guessing your presents. But can you really know things in advance? Or was it just a lucky hunch? Is it real . . . or just coincidence? And what about déjà vu? And how about love at first sight? Your lot, my friend is: Psychic gifts.

ᚹ Ⓥ Ⓦ

Wonder

9 You are **WUNJO**, the happy one. And it's true, I see you with a big grin on your face. I see you winking at me. And to you, it's just a game. What would life be like without a couple of laughs? Might as well get 'em while they're still hot. But what did you come here wishing for? And what did you find instead? Life's a gas, isn't it? Your lot, my friend, is: Have some kicks.

H (H)

Hail

10 You are **HAGALAZ**, the hardened one. And oh, I see you staring back at me. (Don't try to deny it.) I see your eyes. I see you staring me down. What makes you so abso-blipping-lutely sure? Or is it, you're uncertain? And what's that dark cloud hanging over your head? If you did not want to know the truth, then why did you ask? Your lot, my friend, is: Be a cynic.

✝ (N)

Need

11 You are **NAUDHIZ**, the needy one. So I suspect that's you I hear singing the blues. Or is it crossover country? Why all the tears? It's only whining guitars. Haven't you seen your way through plenty already? And won't this surely pass? What's the one thing you need the most of right now? Let's all get in a big circle and say a prayer for it. Your lot, my friend, is: Be a survivor.

I (I)

Ice

12 You are **ISA**, the cold-blooded one. So why do I see your heart melting? Or is it your minds melding? And why do I see you running naked through the snow? Is this what it takes to make you tingle? Or was it just a friendly game of Truth or Dare?[3] How does it feel to expose yourself? (And will you still respect me later?) Your lot, my friend, is: Love 'em or leave 'em.

◇ (Y) (J)

Year

13 You are **JERA**, the successful one. So why do I see you trudging home? Is it just the end of one of those days? Or do you always work this hard? You must be exhausted. How do you do it? Yet what exhil-

---

[3] See Reading #16, Extra Credit section.

aration you must feel at the same time. Isn't it great to have accomplished so much in so short a time? And doesn't your body feel proud? Your lot, my friend, is: Work for your supper.

◻

borderline weird

14 You are **WEIRD**, but only sometimes. Which is why, I suppose, I see you walking a very fine line. What are these occasional "fits" you have? And how can you be so "normal" all the rest of the time? What makes you vacillate so? And why are you standing in the doorway now? Come in, or else go out already. Your lot, my friend, is: Right down the middle.

↸ Ⓔ

hElp

15 You are **EIHWAZ**, the protected one. So no wonder I see a Guardian Angel looking out for you . . . a Spirit Guide, if you will. And don't you try to pooh-pooh it. I know you've seen it work. Or is it just blind luck that's got you through it all so far? Something must be intervening in your life. And it must be for the good. Your lot is this: You get by with a little help from above.

◪ Ⓟ

hoPe

16 You are **PERTHRO**, the charmed one. And I can see you casting Runes like a Viking. They all come naturally to you. But which sign comes up the most for you? And are you surprised you got this one? Don't look to me for advice! Be your own Runester. Your lot, my friend, is this: Wake up and read the tea leaves for yourself.

Ψ Ⓩ

reSIStance

17 You are **ELHAZ**, the blessed one. And well I see the halo round your head like a protective aura. You need but lift a hand to ward off danger. But would it not be as easy to bring harm? How can you be so sure that right is right? and wrong is wrong? And how can you show such restraint? Your lot, my friend, is: By faith alone.

⟨ Ⓢ

Sun & Stars

18 You are **SOWILO**, the constant one. And so, I see you sticking to your course . . . sure, certain, dependable, and true. One could set a clock by you. But can it be just force of habit? Has your routine become your rut? Or is it that you're doing what you're actually supposed to? Would you heed a voice that tells you any different? Your lot, my friend, is: Do it your own way.

↑ Ⓣ

Triumph

19 You are **TIWAZ**, the mighty one. And oh, I see you puffing out your pecs and flexing your 'ceps. I see you gazing in the looking glass. Pretty proud of yourself, are you now? Or is that Adonis stare just the look of surprise at what you have made of yourself? Did you ever think you'd carry your own weight? Your lot, my friend, is: Get the lead out.

Ƀ Ⓑ

Birth

20 You are **BERKANO**, the fertile one. Which is why, I suppose, I see bunnies multiplying all around you. Plant enough seeds, and one of them is sure to take hold. How is it you have so many ideas? And how do you fit them all in? What will it be this time? A boy? Or a girl? And do you want to know in advance? Your lot, my friend, is: Be fruitful and multiply.

M Ⓔ

fEmale

21 You are **EHWAZ**, the wise one. Your spirit is old. And I see you have already lived many useful lifetimes. How else could you know so much? How else could you give such good advice? Or do you read a lot? Your own words ring as true as the utterance from any ancient oracle. Your lot, my friend, is: To read between the lines.

ᛗ Ⓜ

Male

22 You are **MANNAZ**, the industrious one. And I see you getting lots of things done with your time. I see you checking things off your list. But aren't there still as many things to do? things left to see? conquer? discover? How do you fit them all in? When do you feel that you're through? Your lot, my friend, is this: To keep yourself busy.

ᛚ Ⓛ

Love

23 You are **LAGUZ**, the connected one. And I see you floating on your back down the eternal stream. I see you gliding by, supported by unseen hands. Have you no cares in the world? no concerns? Does nothing else matter to you but catching the big wave? Or have you already found the answer? Your lot, my friend, is: XXXO. Kisses, kisses, kisses. Hug.

ᛝ Ⓝ

beING

24 You are **INGWAZ**, the sensual one. So I hope I haven't caught you right out of the shower. Or do you always read Runes in the buff? (Just kidding.) Let me put it this way: I see you being tactile and . . . interactive. But don't you ever get tired? And when do you come up for air? Your lot, my friend, is: Human nature.

✖ ⦿

hOme

25 You are **OTHALA**, the sheltered one. And I see you living safe and sound within your compound. But why have you walled up? And what have you walled in? Is this your dreamworld? your love shack? or just your safety net? Your lot, my friend, is: Home sweet home.

⋈ ⦿

Destiny

26 You are **DAGAZ**, the fulfilled one. I see you going where you need to go. I see you doing what you need to do. I even see you making a name for yourself. And is that you I see smirking right now? It's true then. Don't you already know? Why would you doubt the best news of all? Go on . . . have a wonderful life. Your lot, my friend, is: Show us how it's done.

☐ ☐

weird

27 You are **WEIRD**, the brilliant one. And I see you going your own way through the world. I see you making an eccentric difference. Well, why not? Is God's Universe not diverse? Is there not a place on the ark for two of every kind? Who's to say what's meant? Your lot, my friend, is: Know thine own genius.

EXTRA CREDIT

To assess what's meant to be. Gather your Runes together and mix them up while you think of the issue at hand. Ask your question: **What is the fate of _____?** this project? this career move? this political stand? this investment? our love? Draw the one that feels right to you tonight, and turn it into its upright position. Look it up in this Reading's Answer section. If you draw the Blank Rune, you'll have to choose among the four answers (positions 0, 1, 14, and 27).

EXTRA, EXTRA CREDIT!

To get your thought for the day. Reach into your Runes and feel around until you find the Rune that edges its way into the palm of your hand. Then find your Rune either in this Reading's Answer section or in the Master Answer section at the back of the book. (When using the Master Answer section, consider reversals.)

Go on to the next Reading whenever you are ready to continue.

Reading #24

HOW DO I DO THIS ON MY OWN?
(Abracadabra)

In this Reading you will learn how to improvise with your Runes . . .
how to make up your own questions, define your own rules, and
read your own signs. You can also use this Reading as a quick
review of what you may have picked up from the rest of the book.

◁▷◁▷

RUNE TOOLS

To conduct Readings on your own, you will need a set of Rune
"stones," "staves," "tiles," "lots"—whatever you want to call them. If
you can't find any at the stores, they're fairly easy to make. All you
need is 25 smallish objects, like beach pebbles, poker chips, Popsicle
sticks, wooden nickels, wood chips, twigs . . . just about anything fin-
ger-sized will work. Once you've got your cache of objects assembled,
just write, carve, or paint one letter of the Runic alphabet on each,
leaving one blank. (Consult the Index for a list of Rune-making
activities covered in the book.) Your finished set of Runes will look
like this . . .

ᚠ	ᚷ	ᛄ	ᛗ
ᚢ	ᚹ	ᚲ	ᛘ
ᚦ	ᚺ	ᛉ	ᛚ
ᚨ	ᛏ	ᛊ	ᛤ
ᚱ	ᛁ	ᛋ	ᛟ
ᚲ	ᛃ	ᛒ	ᛗ	☐

319

Or you can also use the English alphabet if you prefer, in which case you'll be working with 29 tiles.[1]

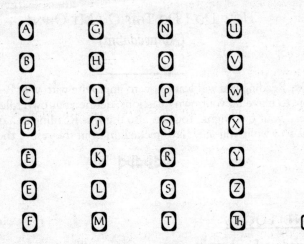

Scrabble® tiles are ideal. To use them, you'll need one of every letter, plus an extra *E* and both blanks. Pencil a "**Th**" on one of the blank tiles and draw a caret over one of the *E*'s. (You might also want to underline your *O* and your *Z* so that you can tell when they are right side up and upside down.)

HOW TO

To consult your Runes, the first thing you need to do is think about what you're interested in finding out. What question would you like help in answering? What's the biggest worry on your mind? What are you trying to decide? What problem has you hog-tied?

How to ask questions. Every oracle has its strength. Runes are best at helping you work your way through issues, problems, and

---

[1] For the benefit of statisticians and other math hounds: With the standard Futhark Runes, the odds are 1 in 25 that you will draw any given letter on a single pick. To approximate these same odds with your alphabet tiles, you can skip the letters *C*, *Q*, *V*, and *J* in your set, since they make the same sounds as the Futhark's **K**, **W**, and **Y**. The odds for your alphabet tiles will now be exactly the same as the Futhark Runes.

concerns. So if you want to learn how to handle situations, relationships, or conditions better, you've come to the right place. Runes are best at answering "what," "how," and sometimes "why" questions.

What should I do about _____?

How can I deal with _____?

Why is so-and-so doing such-and-such?

What is my future with this person? place? or thing?

How are my prospects with regard to _____?

What's the situation with _____?

How will _____ turn out?

But Runes can be quite cooperative and will do their best to answer any question—be it yea or nay . . . who, when, or where. No subject is off-limits, especially if it's private, personal, and confidential. After all, who else can you talk to? And how else will you ever work your way through it?

Work:	What must I do to get ahead?
Career:	How did the interview go?
Love:	How does so-and-so really feel about me?
Sex:	What if we . . . you-know?
Property:	What will sell the house?
Politics:	Will the media buy it?
Finance:	Is this a good investment?
Business:	What's the bottom line?
Religious:	What do You want me to do?
Spiritual:	How can I fulfill my purpose?

However—be advised—if there is a pressing issue that is more important to you right now than the question you asked, the Runes may well choose to tell you about it, instead. Look for subtle messages as well as blatant hints and a few ironic twists.

How to give commands. A neat thing about Runes is, you don't
really have to ask a question at all. Just get the subject clearly in
your mind. Picture the person you are concerned about. Picture the
place you want to know about. Picture the project you are working
on. Picture anything relevant to the issue—as a means of focusing
in on it.

Once you home in on this mental picture, you're ready to select
your Runes. You don't really have to say anything. But in lieu of a
question, at this point you can give your Runes a command:

> **Tell me** about _____.
>
> **Give me** word about _____.
>
> **Reveal** the truth about _____.
>
> **Show** me what to do about _____.

How to use magic words. Interestingly enough, the Runes will also
produce good results if you just say a couple of "magic words." Some
magical expressions used in this book are:

Presto! Chango!	**Mirror, mirror!**
Voilà!	**Double, double!**
Hocus-pocus!	**Pretty please!**
Abracadabra	**Speak!**

It's kind of a fun touch. But you don't really have to say anything
at all. Just keep your topic in mind until you've selected your Runes.
How to Psych Up. If you find you have trouble concentrating, take
a little extra time to prepare for working with your Runes. A nice
hot bath works psychic wonders, as does a cold shower (brr!). To set
the mood, lower the lights. (Runes were typically read in firelight.)
Get yourself a candle. Put on a little mood music. Say a prayer for
guidance if you like. But as far as more elaborate preparations go, it's
really not required. By their very nature, Runes are spontaneous.
They seem to enjoy being done on the fly, on the spur of the
moment, at the drop of a hat.
How many to pick? Once you have decided what you want to know
about, it's time to decide how many Runes you need to draw to get

the answer. Tradition says three. But a single Rune can tell you all you need to know. And two Runes often do the trick. (But three does seem to be the magic number.)

If you select more than three Runes, the answers can start to get vague, contradictory, confusing, or downright overwhelming with detail. However, you can draw as many as five or six with good results. Play around with it and see what works best for you. But when in doubt, default to three.

How to select your Runes. Regardless of how many Runes you decide to pick today, there are two ways to select them. Both are fun and equally effective.

<u>Drawing Runes</u>. One way to consult the Runes is to simply "draw them from your hat."

1 Think of the matter you want to know about while you run your hands through your Runes. Since many people keep their Runes in a cloth bag, all you have to do is reach in and feel around.

2 Or you can spill all of your Runes out on a table or the floor and rustle them, while you focus on your topic.

3 When you have the matter you want to know about fully in mind, ask your question, give a command, say the magic words, or just form a mental picture and . . . grab.

The experience of grabbing a Rune varies from occasion to occasion. Sometimes a Rune will seem to want to worm its way into your hand. Sometimes you will find you have to chase it all over the bag to get hold of it. And sometimes three will leap into your hand all at once. It's most intriguing. Take whatever Rune you latch on to— or that latches on to you. It's generally the right one. And if not, try again. All oracles have been known to glitch, which is one of the things that makes them so charming.

<u>Casting Runes</u>. The other way to select Runes involves throwing them, which is not only traditional, but it's also lots of fun.

1 Just mix up your Runes as before (in the bag or on the floor).

2 With your issue fully in mind, grab a handful (or all of them if you can manage). Shout out your question. Bark your command.

Intone your magic words. Or simply lock in on your mental image. And toss your Runes on the floor or any flat surface.

3 Now—without peeking—reach into this pile and grab one, two, three, or however many you decided in advance to use.

How to turn over your Runes. As you select each Rune, you need to be a little careful what you do with it. Every Rune has a front side (ᚠ ᚢ ᚦ ᚱ ᚲ ᚲ) and a flip side (◻ ◻ ◻ ◻ ◻ ◻). To see which Rune you've drawn, sometimes you're going to have to turn it over so that you can see the Rune on the back. And here's where you have to be a tad careful . . .

Every Rune also has a standard, upright position (ᚠ ᚢ ᚦ ᚻ ᚱ ᚲ). But many of them look different when they are viewed upside down (ᛆ ᚿ ᚵ ᚼ ᛣ ᛞ). These reversed Runes have slightly different meanings from their upright counterparts. The point is, depending on how you turn your Rune over in your hand when you go to look at it, you may inadvertently change an upright Rune into a reversed Rune.

There's nothing wrong in drawing a reversed Rune, of course, but it <u>will</u> make a difference in how you interpret the answer. I maintain that if you were supposed to flip the Rune over in the process of selecting it, you will. So, in general, don't worry about it. To avoid unintentional reversals, turn your Runes from side to side: ◻ ➜ ᚠ or ◻ ➜ ᚪ, rather from top to bottom: ◻ ↓ ᚪ If you still feel the answer you're getting is not quite right, consult both the upright and reversed meanings.

How to line up your Runes. As you select each Rune, turn it Rune-side up, and place it in front of you, starting from the left and moving right.

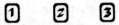

If you prefer, you can do it backhanded, right to left. Either way is traditional and appropriate.

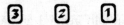

324

There are various ways to define each of these three positions. And there are several other Rune layouts that you can use. Consult the Quick Reference Guide for more details. But in general, all that's left to do at this point is interpret your answer.

THE ANSWERS

By their built-in magic, your 25 Runes or 29 alphabet tiles have the potential to give you up to 40 different answers on a single draw. The secret to this Runic dynamic is that most (but not all) of the letters look distinctly different upside down.

If you are working with the Futhark Runes, the 40 possible answers are these:

1	ᚠ	13	ᚷ	20	ᛃ	30	ᛗ
2	ᚡ					31	ᛘ
3	ᚢ	14	ᚱ	21	ᚲ	32	ᛙ
4	ᚣ	15	ᚴ	22	ᛈ	33	ᛚ
5	ᚤ	16	ᚺ	23	ᛉ	34	ᛁ
6	ᚥ			24	ᛇ	35	ᛂ
7	ᚦ	17	ᛏ	25	ᛋ	36	ᛞ
8	ᚧ						
9	ᚨ	18	ᛁ	26	ᛏ	37	ᛝ
10	ᚩ			27	ᛐ	38	ᛟ
11	ᚪ	19	ᛊ	28	ᛒ	39	ᛠ
12	ᚫ			29	ᛓ		
						40	☐

By current practice and long-standing tradition, the Runes that look just alike upright and upside down have no reversed meanings. Counting the Blank Rune, there are 10 of them. Depending on how your Runes are positioned on your tiles, some of these may actually look reversed to you. But—to prove my point—these Runes, which were centered on their tiles by a computer, are virtually indistinguishable right side up and upside down: ⊠ ⊠, ᛜ ᛜ, ✛ ✛, ⸾ ⸾, ⧖ ⧖, ↕ ↕, ⊂ ⊃, ⋈ ⋈, ⋈ ⋈.

If you are working with alphabet tiles, the concept is the same, but to achieve the same dynamic, we sometimes double-up a couple of English letters that make the same sound in Runes. And to account for the fact that some English letters can be reversed, but can't be in Runes, we sometimes double them up too. Here's how your alphabet tiles work to produce 40 answers . . .

1 F	13 G G	20 E E	30 E
2 Ⅎ			31 Ǝ
3 U	14 V W	21 P	32 M
4 Ո	15 Λ M	22 d	33 W
5 Th	16 H	23 Z	34 L
6 ꓩ		24 Z	35 ⅃
7 A	17 N	25 S	36 X
8 Ɐ			
9 R	18 I	26 T	37 O
10 ꓤ		27 Ⱶ	38 O
11 C K Q	19 Y ⅄	28 B	39 D ꓷ
12 Ɔ ꓘ Ò	J ꓩ	29 ꓭ	40 ▯

The main trick to using alphabet tiles is that you need to distinguish between upright and reversed versions of the Z-Rune and the O-Rune, which (in English) don't look much different right side up and upside down. Hopefully your letter tiles will be like my alphabet fonts, and you will be able to tell them apart, based on their position on the tile: ⌐Z ⌐Z, ⌐O ⌐O. If not, pencil a line underneath the letter to represent its upright version. Okay, with that caveat, you're all set.

To interpret your answers. Start by looking up each Rune in the Quick Reference Guide's Master Answer section.

The answers appear in the traditional order of the Runes,[2] with reversed Runes immediately following their upright counterparts:

F̂	U	Th	A	R	K	G	W	H	N	I	Y
Ê	P	Z	S	T	B	E	M	L	X	O	D ⌐

K=C & Q; W=V; Y=J

The Master Answer section includes a general description for each Rune, with specific interpretations for Work, Love, Money, and Strategy questions. Read the entire description for your Rune (upright or reversed). Or just focus on that portion of the text that relates to your question. The Strategy section will generally answer questions that are not readily classified into one of the other categories.

These answers are meant to help you form your own interpretations. The text may be right-on tonight. Or you may have to read between the lines a bit, pick up a key word here and there, and surmise the rest. In general, don't take them too literally. The important thing is that you take away from these brief descriptions what you need. Look for the larger message. (I often find that the questions I hear myself asking are equally as informative as the answers!)

---

[2] There is some controversy as to whether O comes before D, or D comes before O. I have opted for the sequence shown, based on the work of R. I. Page, professor of Anglo-Saxon at the University of Cambridge.

You may also find that Readings #17, #18, and #19, which include pictures for each Rune, are useful for general purpose readings.

Come what may, don't hesitate to draw your own conclusions. Make up your own mind. Reach your own decisions. And—God willing—the destiny that is yours alone to build will become clearer with the help of these mere Runes.

Good luck, my friend.

Quick
Reference Guide
to the Runes
and
their Meanings

Rune Layouts

Before reading this section, you might want to review Reading #24, which explains how to ask questions of the Runes and describes the basic techniques for drawing and casting them. When conducting your own Readings, it's up to you to decide how many Runes you need for a particular question. It's also up to you to decide how you're going to line them up in a layout or spread. This section reviews some of the more popular spreads you could use.

One-Rune Draws

It only takes a single Rune to give you an answer. In fact, simple one-Rune draws are an excellent way to begin every session with your Runes.

HOW TO

Mix up your Runes while you think about the issue you're facing. Ask your question, give your command, say the magic word, or say nothing at all. Then cast a handful of Runes on the floor and pick one. Or reach into your bag and select the one that feels right today. Note whether it is upright or reversed. Then look it up in the Master Answer section. Read the whole text that goes with your Rune or focus in on the Work, Love, Money, or Strategy sections.

TIPS

In general, a single Rune will describe the situation you are in. But in many cases, it also carries some advice. For a demonstration of one-Rune draws, turn to Reading #1, #2, or #3. Or check out the Extra Credit section of Reading #18 ("Run interference for me") or the Extra, Extra Credit Section of Reading #15 ("Double, double, take my trouble").

TWO-RUNE PICKS

By selecting two Runes instead of one, you will start to add detail and depth to your own readings. The second Rune you pick tends to show the challenge that greets you. Together with the situation described by the first, you begin to assemble the information you need to develop an action plan.

HOW TO

With your issue in mind, mix up your Runes. Ask your question. Cast a handful of Runes on the floor and grab one. Or reach into your bag and select the Rune that comes into your hand. Place your Rune faceup in front of you. Then reach into the Runes you have thrown (or into your bag) and select one more. Place it to the right of the Rune you drew first:

Or you can place it to the left, it makes no difference, as long as you remember the order in which you picked them. Look up each Rune in the Master Answer section and read the entire text or only the portions that are directly relevant to your question or issue.

TIPS

In interpreting your answers, remember that the first Rune you chose describes the current situation, and the second describes something that represents a challenge. However, it's also possible that the two Runes taken together will just form a continuous thought. In which case, take the message for what it's worth.

VARIATIONS

Check out Readings #11 through #16, in which Rune pairs are used to learn about yourself and the others in your life. For an interesting diversion, Reading #17's Extra Credit section uses a two-Rune draw to compute odds. Or play a game of Truth or Dare in Reading #16.

THREE-RUNE SPREADS

The traditional way to read Runes is three at a time. And three-Rune spreads are the primary method used in *Runes in Ten Minutes*. It's a simple, straightforward technique that will mold to fit just about any question you put to it.

HOW TO

With your topic in mind, mix up the Runes in your bag. Ask your question. Give a command. Or say your magic words. Draw three Runes, one at a time. Or toss a handful of Runes on the floor and select three. Line them up, Rune side up in front of you, left to right . . .

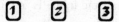

. . . or right to left if you prefer: **3**, **2**, **1**. Then look up each Rune (upright or reversed) in the Master Answer section.

TIPS

In interpreting your Runes, the context for your answers comes from the meaning that you attach to each position in the three-Rune lay-out. If you don't define them otherwise in advance, the Runes will generally default to these settings:

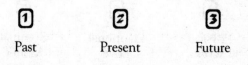

1   **2**   **3**

Past   Present   Future

But most spreads can just as easily be read as:

Situation Challenge Outcome

The Extra, Extra Credit section of Reading #3 demonstrates the basic idea.

VARIATIONS

The three positions can be set to just about any three things you can think of. Some variations on the basic theme are:

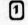

Situation	Action	Result
Strength	Weakness	Outcome
Force	Counterforce	Resolution

Putting things into a time frame is often useful. Just "set" your layout to work like a clock. . . .

Yesterday	Today	Tomorrow
Last Year	This Year	Next Year
Start	Middle	Finish

You can also program your spread to answer a question on three different levels at once:

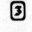

Physical	Emotional	Spiritual
Work	Love	Money
Step 1	Step 2	Step 3

Or—here's a wacky idea!—you don't even have to define them at all. To see what I mean, just try out the Extra Credit sections of Reading #8, #12, #13, or #21.

Thor's Cross

Once you've mastered the basic techniques, you might like to move ahead to an interesting five-Rune spread, named in honor of the same Norse god who lent us his name for "Thursday."

HOW TO

Get your issue in mind while you mix up your Runes. Ask your question or give your command. Reach in your bag and select five Runes, one at a time, and place them in this formation:

```
        ⁴
  ¹  ²  ³
        ⁵
```

Or cast a big handful of Runes on the floor and select five. Look up each Rune (upright or reversed) in the Master Answer section.

TIPS

As with the three-Rune spread, how you interpret your five-Rune spread is dependent on how you defined each of the positions of the layout in advance. If you don't define them otherwise, they default as follows: Rune 1 is the past. Rune 2 is the present. Rune 3 is the future. Rune 4 is what you can change. And Rune 5 is what you can't change.

VARIATIONS

There are other ways both to construct and interpret the Thor's Cross layout. One that is very similar to a standard Tarot spread looks like this:

In this case, the positions stand for: 1) the present situation; 2) the best you can hope for; 3) the experience you need to draw upon; 4) A recent development; and 5) the future outcome.

Runes in Ten Minutes uses a variation of Thor's Cross in the Extra Credit sections of Readings #14 and #15 in order to trace the developments associated with love affairs and friendships.

For general purposes, you can interpret this layout using the same positon definitions listed above.

These are only some of the possibilities for using this versatile spread. Feel free to lay out Thor's Cross in the way that feels most natural and comfortable to you. You can also experiment with the meanings assigned to each position in the spread. The Runes will adapt to most any definition you place on the various positions of any layout.

Master Answer Section

For full instructions, see Reading #24. The answers appear in the traditional order of the Runes, with reversed Runes immediately following their upright counterparts. Ten Runes (✕, ዘ, ✝, ᛁ, ◇, ↑, ≤, ▨, ⋈, and ◻) have no reversals.

F U Th A R K G W H N I Y Ê P Z S T B E M L X O D

ᚠ ᚢ ᚦ ᚨ ᚱ ᚲ ᚷ ᚹ ᚺ ᛁ ◇ ↑ ᛃ ᛦ ᛊ ᛏ ᛒ ᛖ ᛗ ᛚ ⋈ ⋈ ⋈

◻ The Blank Rune appears last. K=C & Q; W=V; Y=J

ᚠ Ⓕ

Fortune

F is for "Fortune." *Say the word!* The F-Rune is about the power of money. You have buying power, spending power, borrowing power, and lending power. This is a material world, to be sure. Money, real estate, personal property, and material assets of all kinds are up for grabs. But how will you attract such things? And once you've got them, what will they do for you? People of affluence and influence are involved. Beware! Some will surely attempt to use you for personal gain. Yet another enemy resides within. How much does it take to keep you satisfied? And what price are you willing to pay to keep it all in operating condition? Money *is* power. But it is also freedom, if that's what you choose to buy with it. *Traditional names: Fehu, The Cattle. The Things a Person Possesses. The Things We Value. A Beast of Burden.*

For WORK questions. Salary, perqs, and benefits! All right, who's been bucking for a bonus? Looks like you can expect a little something extra on deposit come payday. Or maybe I could show you something in a window office? Somebody gives you a little pat on the back (but don't take it too personally).

For LOVE questions. Money is no object! So, Mama, order anything on the menu. And hey, Pop, spring for the bottle with a cork. Wining and dining is in order—even if you have to put it on plastic.

Love has no price, of course. And sex is never free. So—what say?—should I put you down for the limo? Or would you rather take a moonlit stroll? Someone spares no expense.

For MONEY questions. A mark, a yen, a buck, or a pound! Let's see, at today's conversion rates, compounded over several years, and net, net . . . it looks like a sure bet to me. You might even see an early return if you're lucky. But for best results, stick with it for the long haul. Take stock of liquid assets. Watch your cash flow. Count your receipts.

For STRATEGY questions. Inventory! In general, the situation is fortuitous. All you have to do is look at the books to see for yourself. Count and appraise your possessions. Assess net present value. But put the focus on long-term assets. Accumulate wealth.

◢ 🄵

Fortune reversed

F is for "Fortune." *Say the word!* Reversed, the **F**-Rune is about the power to reverse your fortune . . . for better or worse. The good news is, things that spiral down generally rise back up again. That which is temporarily depleted can usually be restocked. And besides, everything is relative. On the downside, things might get worse before they get better. But it's also possible you've bottomed out already, and the tides are just about to turn back to your favor. Either way, you have the wherewithal to ride out this economic downturn. And if you're lucky, you might even come out of it all the richer in the end. One thing's for certain: It's a small price to pay for the big lesson it brings. *Traditional names: Fehu reversed, The Cattle. Lost or Stolen Property. Bartered Goods. Liquidated Assets. A Person of Few Means. The Things that Possess You.*

For WORK questions. Companies changing hands! Something has either been sold off or bought out. There are new owners. And with them come fresh managers with bottom-line ideas. Costs are cut. Quality is sacrificed. There may even be a reduction in force. Work longer hours if you have to. Do the job of several if you must. It's a bear, I know. But you can turn it around.

For LOVE questions. Two can live as cheaply! (And there is a sizable tax advantage.) Well, when you're in love, spaghetti is romantic. A little Chianti, and who knows? But if you've been fighting over money, join the club. Let's have everybody cut back a little and see if we can make these ends meet. It's only for a little while. Besides, it'll be fun. We'll make a game of it.

For MONEY questions. Due diligence! It's not the time for acting without thinking . . . but then again, when is? Shop around for the best bargain. Inspect the goods before you buy. And make sure you understand the terms and conditions before you sign on the dotted line.

For STRATEGY questions. Make the most of it! So it's not the best of times, Charlie. It's not the worst of times, either. You might as well look upon it as a "challenge." Call it what you will. Just don't throw up your hands in despair. For there is much to be accomplished here. You need to turn things around to your favor. Put the **F**-Rune in your pocket and say your magic words. Then roll up your sleeves and get to the task.

⋀ ⓤ

lUck

U is for "lUck." *Say the word!* The **U**-Rune is about the power of luck to stick with you. There are things that go out of their way to go right for you. And there are things that go out of their way to keep <u>you</u> from going wrong. But is your horseshoe pointed up or down? Your luck is yours alone, my friend. And it's your friend for life. So by now you know what kind of luck clings to you and what kind does not adhere. You can always hold out hope that some new charm will do the trick. But this is one of those times when the sort of luck you have as a rule continues to hold true in general. One thing is for sure: You can thank your lucky stars right now, because something is about to drop in your lap. Or else, you are about to avoid a close scrape. *Traditional names: Uruz, The Wild Ox. Aurochs—The Beast of the Forest Primeval. The Untamed and Untamable Creature. A Free Spirit.*

For WORK questions. Lucky break! Things couldn't have worked out better if you'd planned it. You squeak by again, or else sail through with flying colors—whichever is your way. And don't it make you wonder? Job offers, promotions, raises, bonuses, and commendations are favored. But the important thing is that you get to keep on being paid. Everything's going to be okay.

For LOVE questions. Lucked out! Your eyes met . . . locked . . . and something passed between you—two ships and all that. Or else, you happened to bump into each other again and took it as a sign. Does it really matter who made the first move? You did what you did. And you know what you know. The lucky part is intuitively obvious.

For MONEY questions. Manna from heaven! It seems like when you need it, cash comes. You earn some. You borrow some. You win some. Some gets refunded. Some gets reimbursed. It's as if someone is keeping an eye out for you. It's as if someone is looking out for you. You've always got enough to get by on. And that's damn lucky.

For STRATEGY questions. Keep your fingers crossed! This situation requires you to have luck on your side. Things either need to go your way, or else you need to get out of their way as they go wrong. There's not much else to do besides wear your lucky cap. But from under your brim, keep your eyes peeled for developments of both kinds.

⋀ ⋂

lUck reversed

U is for "lUck." *Say the word!* The **U**-Rune reversed is about the power to attract good luck and repel bad luck. How shall I nail up your horseshoe, then? Prongs up to capture the good stuff? Or prongs down to ward off the crap? Take your pick. Make your statement. (The nails are lucky, too, by the way.) But—as the old saying goes—be careful what you wish for. Also be careful what you wish not. That which might appear at first blush as misfortune can just as easily turn out to be the luckiest thing that ever happened to you. And that which at first glance seems to be a blessing may yet prove to have its curse. *Traditional names: Uruz reversed, The Wild Ox. The Extinct Beast of the Wilderness. That Which Has Gone Away. The Broken Spirit.*

For WORK questions. Tough luck! Sorry 'bout that, pal. But you see it's only business and nothing personal. Just get everything you've got coming before you hit the road. And don't slam any doors, especially the ones that are already closed. Kiss them on the cheek good-bye. Accept the luck they wish you.

For LOVE questions. Love sucks! Why do these things always happen to you? (Poor baby!) Well, heck, you can always cry on my shoulder. But better yet, rip out a Scratch Pad and dry your eyes. It was good while it lasted, wasn't it? And there are plenty more fish in the sea. Maybe you just need a different lure. Here's a little love charm you can use: ✱.[1]

For MONEY questions. The tintinnabulation of the bills! Wow! Is that all your mail? And what's this pink one? Well there's only one thing to do. And it involves two saints with names beginning with P. You may, indeed, have to rob Peter to pay Paul. But at any rate, you either need more income or less expense. For starters, perhaps you could cut back on lottery tickets? How about a friendly game of Scrabble® instead?

For STRATEGY questions. Get lucky! The situation requires you to turn a stint of hard times into better days. It's time to take the bull by the nose, horns, or other vital parts. Start by carrying the U-Rune around in your pocket as a confidence booster. Every time your hand crosses it, think positive thoughts. Imagine things turning out right. Then take appropriate action to see that they do just that. Good luck!

ᚠ Ⓣⱨ

faiTh

Th is for "fai**Th**." *Say the word!* The **Th**-Rune is about the power of positive believing. So whatever fate befalls you, remember: You

---

[1] ✱ is a Runic symbol that signifies eternal love. See Reading #12's Extra, Extra Credit section for instructions on how to make a love charm.

always have the option of calling on your God. And everything will be better, as long as you believe . . . hard enough . . . long enough . . . firm enough . . . true enough. And as long as you ask earnestly and in the right way. If it seems like a lot of conditions, well, that's what religion is . . . and politics and science and medicine and metaphysics and whatever else you choose to put your faith in. Just be a little careful about buying off on all of anything. There's money and power politics everywhere you look. And few things are exactly as they seem. But if you can't trust your own faith, then what can you believe in? *Traditional names: Thurisaz, The Thorn. Whitethorn. Blackthorn. The Forest Undergrowth. A Strong One. A Vexing One. The Giant at the Top of the Beanstalk.*

For WORK questions. Let us bow our heads! Your religion is your work. Your work is your religion. But you will have to tell me what that means, exactly. Because if you're counting on the owners and stockholders to take care of you later, I'd advise counting again. Faith is a valuable thing to place. Reserve it for those who deserve it. When in doubt, pray for the good sense to tell the difference.

For LOVE questions. Keeping only unto each other! Your vows are involved, my friend. The question is, what did you agree to? Haven't you been faithful so far? Aren't you good to your word? And do you have any cause to doubt your partner? A pledge is a pledge. Plight each other your troth. And may I have the ring, please? If need be, seal it again with a kiss.

For MONEY questions. Lilies of the field! They never worry. And neither should you. Their God is looking out for them. And so is yours, for you. But perhaps a little offering is in order. Cough up a couple of bucks for the hungry children of the world. And don't forget to render unto Caesar every April the 15th.

For STRATEGY questions. Light a candle! The situation requires you to invoke powers greater than your own. So put on your cloak and hood and step into the magic circle. Or else, cover your head and kneel down at the rail. Bow to the east if you're so inclined. Ring a bell. Bang a drum. Open your prayer book to the invocation. And in a moment of silence, state your heartfelt wish.

◀ ⑨

faiTh reversed

Th is for "fai**Th**." *Say the word!* The **Th**-Rune reversed is about the power of negative believing. So I'd say something has caused you to doubt what you once regarded as God's Honest Truth. Or else, part of your accepted faith requires you to deny, doubt, or denounce certain other beliefs. No one has a corner on the market for truth, of course. And every system has its strengths as well as its weaknesses. Take what you need and leave the rest, I guess. But if you're going to mix and match, be prepared for potluck. And if you must give something up to get in The Spiritual Club, just make sure it's not your library. *Traditional names: Thurisaz reversed, The Thorn. A Burr in Your Side. Something that Needles at You. Inner Doubts.*

For WORK questions. Switch jobs! The old place just isn't cutting it. You've grown tired of the whole cast of characters and weary of dealing with the same old situations again and again and again. It was time to move on anyway. Look for people you can trust . . . and something you can believe in.

For LOVE questions. Change partners! Allemande left, do-si-do . . . and all that square-dance stuff. What exactly have you been up to in your (ahem) free time? Looks like the old flame just wasn't cutting it. Or do you make a habit of this? If things are starting to get dull at home, how about changing roles?

For MONEY questions. In God we trust! And when it comes to truth in accounting, God's about the only one I would recommend putting your trust in. If something has happened to cause you to doubt the sincerity of a business partner or financial institution, request a full accounting.

For STRATEGY questions. Suspend your disbelief! The situation you are in requires you to put your rational, scientific, and objective thoughts on hold. For this is a question of belief. It's time to put your faith to the acid test. Take the cola challenge, my friend.

ᚠ Ⓐ

fAte

A is for "fAte." *Say the word!* The **A**-Rune is about the power of words to alter the tide of events . . . change the course of history . . . and turn the wheel of fate. But whether this is a time for formal speeches or casual remarks, only you can decide. But I think there's something you've been meaning to tell someone. My friend, the floor is yours. Just be yourself. Share your thoughts. Express your feelings. Get things off your chest. Say what's on your mind. And better yet, relate what you've learned. Hand things down. What can it hurt? And who knows, you might even change the way things go. *Traditional names: Ansuz, The Mouth. That Which Speaks. A Word that Is Voiced. An Idea Come to Life. Poetry in Motion.*

For WORK questions. Speak up! They can't hear you from the executive tower. (Perhaps that's the general idea.) But don't let distance stop you from expressing your ideas. Just be sure to package it in a way The Suits can relate to. This is business, after all. You hold your fate in your own hands . . . and the future is built on buzz words.

For LOVE questions. Whisper sweet nothings! It's a night for romance. So lower your voice as well as the lights. Haul out your favorite volume of poems. Put on some love songs, and hold each other close. Or else take a walk. Talk things over. And when the moment is right, pop your question. From here on out, everything is different.

For MONEY questions. Say when! It looks like your money's doing the talking. But what's it saying about you? Enough's enough already. It's time to speak both dollars and sense. Count all the beans correctly and be sure all the totals tie out. Draw charts and graphs to plot your plight. Then put some words around it. The past has passed. But the future's what you make it out to be.

For STRATEGY questions. Make your case! The situation requires you to talk your way into something, out of something, or through something. At any rate, it is your words that will determine the outcome. So choose carefully, but don't get hung up on them.

Outline the points you want to make. Go over it in your head. But in the end, use the words that fall naturally from your lips.

↓ Ⓥ

fAte reversed

A is for "fAte." *Say the word!* Or else, say nothing at all, I guess. The A-Rune reversed is about the power of silence to change the way things go. So is your silence, then, consent? Or do you mean it as a warning? Know this: Some cannot read between the lines so well. And if you bite your tongue too hard, it may hurt you in the morning. What do your inner voices tell you to do? Speak now or forever hold your peace? Or is it that, in denying them your thoughts, you hope to send a louder message? And is it getting through? Think once more before you speak. *Traditional names: Ansuz reversed, The Mouth. The Words of the Ancestors. Common Sense. Folk Wisdom. The Lessons of History. Spirit Voices.*

For WORK questions. Put up or shove off! What can I say? When you depend on that paycheck, they've got you by the Runes. Better keep your mouth shut—at least for a little while. And if it's a matter of principle, well, you know where the door is.

For LOVE questions. Silent partners! So what's the big secret? Or is it that silence is golden? The two of you don't seem to be communicating. Well, you don't have to talk all the time to have a good relationship. But if there's something you've been meaning to say, quit biting your lip.

For MONEY questions. Hushed money! All I can say is, you must be involved in a deal that's better not to discuss openly—at least not until the public announcement is ready. Perhaps it's a hot tip? Whatever, it's best to keep it to yourself for a while.

For STRATEGY questions. Silence is golden! The situation finds you keeping quiet. Perhaps there is nothing useful or constructive to be said. So you might as well mull it all over. Incubate the idea overnight. Stew in your own juices, if you like. They can wait for your reply in the morning. It never hurts to leave a pregnant pause.

ᚱ Ⓡ

Reality

R is for "Reality." *Say the word!* The **R**-Rune is about the power to create your own reality . . . and to discover your own version of The Truth. But remember now, you're under oath. It's time to be honest with yourself. See it for what it is. Tell it as it is. And call it by its real name. In your own words, please. What is your version of reality? Is it a bed of roses? Or does it suck raw eggs? Even nothing adds up to something by the end of the day. It all depends on your point of view. If you don't know by now what I mean, you'd best go looking some more. Perhaps you'd like a little time alone— or maybe a change of scene. It's not so much where you're going, but how you get there that teaches you. It's time to hit the road. *Traditional names: Raidho, The Journey. A Rough Ride on Horseback. The Search for Wisdom. Forty Days in the Wilderness.*

For WORK questions. Business travel! So all the hotshots have gone off into the woods again, huh? And what newfangled slogans will they bring back this time? Or else, you're about to hit the road yourself. Some business cannot be conducted by phone, fax, or mail. Besides, it's good to get away from it all.

For LOVE questions. Weekend for two! Grab your toothbrush and a change of undies, darlin', because the car's outside idling. Would you rather see the mountains or the beach? A romantic invitation drops into your lap. And everything else is more or less spontaneous. Come Monday, you'll know much more.

For MONEY questions. Traveler's checks! Wherever it is you're going, you'll need some spending money. So don't forget your wallet. Negotiable instruments are involved. Funds may need to be transferred from one account to another. You may need to secure a reservation with your credit card. Be sure to book in advance.

For STRATEGY questions. Wanderlust! The situation involves you in a trip of some kind. There is a place you are coming from. There is a place you're going to. And it's clear you are moving on. Well, they say life itself is a journey. You might as well pack your bag, and chase your dream.

↰ ⟨ℝ⟩

Reality reversed

R is for "**R**eality." *Say the word!* The **R**-Rune reversed is about the power to change your outlook and modify your attitude. Why is it you return from your vacation feeling like a whole new person? And what on earth did you do to your hair? (I guess you had to be there.) It's like glancing in a rearview mirror: Everything behind you is backwards. And it's time now to put things in their proper perspective. Let the feeling linger for a day or two. But then it's back on down to earth for you. Someone is glad to see you return to your home, your job, your faith, your spouse, your family, yourself, or whatever it is you were trying to get away from for a while. I hope you took lots of pictures. *Traditional names: Raidho reversed, The Journey. The Journey's End. The Return from a Trip. The End of a Spiritual Quest.*

For WORK questions. Back to the grindstone! So how was the convention? Or what did you accomplish on the road? Well, write it all up and send it to the files. Turn in your expenses. And if there's any time left in the day, leave messages on other people's voice mail. It's funny how fast it piles up in the electronic in-box. How did they ever get along without you?

For LOVE questions. The honeymoon's over! Alas, all good things must run their course and come to their natural end. But at least maybe now you can get a peaceful night's rest. Unfortunately, there's shaving cream on the towels now or stockings drying in the shower stall. And the hotel maid does not make house calls. Ah, it'll just take a little getting used to and a little getting over the initial shock.

For MONEY questions. Return on investment! An asset appreciates or a deal pays off. And good for you, my friend. But don't forget about capital gains tax and early withdrawal penalties. It might be best to roll it all over into some kind of shelter . . . that is, after you throw it all up in the air and let it rain down on you awhile.

For STRATEGY questions. Come back to your senses! You're in a situation that has a surreal quality about it. Things that are too good to be true, generally are. But it doesn't hurt to wallow in your dreams for a moment. If you need help sorting reality from illusion, place the **R**-Rune in your pocket as a reminder that The Truth resides within you.

< ⊂ Ⓚ ⊙

Course, Quest, Karma

C is for "Course." **Q** is for "Quest." **K** is for "Karma." *Say the words!* The **C**-Rune is about the power to cast light on a subject . . . to understand where it is you're coming from . . . to see clearly where it is you're going to . . . and to shape your own destiny along the way. But don't be surprised if it happens in a sudden, near-blinding flash, like a camera going off inside your head. Passing thoughts form into a "sudden" realization. What is it you've been looking for? Well, here it comes at last. All the pieces fit together now. And in this moment of inspiration you get your payback for all the thought and effort you've expended in the past. Your situation becomes clear now. And all your decisions are made for you. Just follow the bouncing ball. Keep your eye on the light. It's good karma. *Traditional names: Kenaz, The Light. The Torch that Lights the Way. The Beacon Fire. The Forge. The Pyre.*

For WORK questions. Shed some light on the subject! Now's your big chance to shine, my friend. Because somebody wants to hear what you think of things. So drag out your big, bright idea for the future. Generate a couple of computer slides. But mostly tell it as you see it. Give them the benefit of your vision in as few words as possible. Hit the highlights.

For LOVE questions. The light of your life! She was a vision of womanhood. He was a healthy specimen of a man. And together, the two of you sparked the night with light, heat, and smoke. To say anything more would be indiscreet. But let me put it this way: It's good to see you looking so radiant of late.

For MONEY questions. Money to burn! I know that you've been trying to be careful with your cash. But this is one of those times when it's burning a hole in your pocket. The object that is destined to be yours will draw you to it. All you have to do is follow your footsteps to the glow it emits. Will that be paper or plastic? Lucky you, it's probably even on sale.

For STRATEGY questions. Head for the light! The situation you are in requires you to know a good thing when you see it. A knock comes at the door, but only you can tell whether it is a real opportunity or just a sales pitch. An idea comes into your head—but does it last the night? There is, indeed, a light at the end of the tunnel. If you haven't seen it yet, clear your head and wait.

> ◈ Ⓥ ◈

Course, Quest, Karma reversed

C is for "Course." **Q** is for "Quest." **K** is for "Karma." *Say the words!* The **C**-Rune reversed is about the power of darkness . . . to conceal, to heal, and even to reveal in its own way. From the dim recesses of the mind come the deepest thoughts. But turn down the lights first. It's easier to concentrate in a dark, still room. Things come through the hushed light as if in a dream. And it is easier to hear yourself think. In illness too, it helps to draw the shades. For darkness has a way of nurturing both the seed that struggles and the root that stretches deep. It is a comfort also, especially for those who tend to look inside themselves—as you do now. Surely you have come in search of light. Yet your path leads you to this dark spot, where you must sit and cogitate awhile. A candlelit bath might help you sort things out. *Traditional names: Kenaz reversed, The Light. The Light of Reason. Intelligence. The Spark of an Idea.*

For WORK questions. Moonlighting! For some reason you've got to make maximum use of the hours between dusk and dawn. It's even possible you need to take a second job. Or else the current one is the work of two. Okay, then—be that way. But if you're going to work this hard, make sure you save the midnight hour for your love.

For LOVE questions. Lights out! I take it that you're just a tad shy? Or maybe it's that you haven't been getting enough sleep. It couldn't possibly be that you think you have something to hide? Perhaps you just like anonymity?

For MONEY questions. Gray areas! Looks like your time in the think tank paid off. You've found a tax loophole or at least a variation in generally accepted accounting principles that lets you get away with fiscal brilliance. Good for you.

For STRATEGY questions. Sequester yourself! The situation you are in requires you to spend some time in solitary confinement, as it were. There is something blocking your progress that only privacy and isolation can cure. You get your energy from being alone now. For maximum effect, sit silently in darkness for a while.

✗ ☺ ☺

Gifts

G is for "Gifts." *Say the word!* The G-Rune is about the power of gift giving. But are these the gifts you were given? Or the ones you give back? Say it, write it, sing it, or act it out. You can even dance if you like. And if you've got a sixth (or seventh) sense, why waste it? There are as many art forms in the world as there are combinations of Runes and ways to read them. The important thing is that you take the time to express yourself. Practice your craft. Master your art. And don't forget to play around. By combining known skills with secret talents, you define your own gift. And once you've found it, it is yours alone to give. Someone has a gift idea for you. Try not to look it in the mouth. *Traditional names: Gebo, The Gift. A Formal Exchange of Gifts. A Gift for the Host or Hostess. A Housewarming Present. A Diplomatic Gesture.*

For WORK questions. Give it all you've got! It's not creativity they're looking for, you know. But if you package it as innovation, they are sure to respond. The important thing is that you get the job done. Look for ways to improve productivity and profits in your spare time. Donate some personal energy and await your bonus.

For LOVE questions. May I have the ring! Well, I don't know what you had to do to have this gift showered upon you. But it must have been good. And I'm not saying it's a diamond, mind you. But it sure does glitter like gold. A little token of the affections goes a long way to the heart. And don't forget, true value is sentimental, even these days.

For MONEY questions. Give me five! A little birthday money gets doled out. Or an unexpected package comes in the mail.

Perhaps it's Christmas? (Hanukkah? A birthday? Or graduation?) At any rate, the gift wrap is unrolling. And the bows are being tied off. Happy whatever! What do you think you got? And what are you going to do with it?

For **STRATEGY** *questions*. Use your gifts! You're in a situation that requires you to perform up to your potential. So do the best you can on the budget you've got. And if you must spring for a present, make it something tasteful. How about a big smile, for starters?

▶ Ⓥ Ⓦ

Wonder

W is for "Wonder." *Say the word!* The **W**-Rune is about the power of laughter to raise your spirits and the power of joy to warm the cockles of your heart. All of a sudden something tickles you, and a tense situation turns into a moment of comic relief. A joke breaks the ice. A funny story forms the opening remarks. Sometimes you even have to chuckle at yourself. Well, go ahead, then. They say laughter's the best medicine, especially when it comes to healing old wounds. Look at the world around you as if you had not seen it all before, and you will see it as one big surprise after another. Your life right now must be one big barrel of chuckles. Someone sure wants to see if they can make you laugh. *Traditional names: Wunjo, The Joy. Wonder. Glory. Goodwill. Well-being.*

For **WORK** *questions*. Whistle while you work! Heigh-ho. Heigh-ho. It's off to work you go. Or is this a federal holiday? It's nice to hear you arriving in the morning. It's nice to send you off at night. But mostly it's refreshing to see someone who likes the work so much. (And then, of course, there's payday to put a smile on everyone's face.)

For **LOVE** *questions*. Tickle my funny bone! Is that a feather I see behind your back? Or has the cat swallowed the canary again? The two of you are always good for a laugh. (Last night I thought I even heard giggling coming from your room.) It must be time for a celebration of some sort. What else could possibly have put you in such a good mood?

For MONEY questions. Laugh all the way to the bank! Is that money jingling in your pockets? Or is it the bells on your toes? Your step is light these days, as if you haven't a care in the world. Funny what a bank balance will do for a person . . . especially if it's all yours. I guess you showed them, didn't you?

For STRATEGY questions. Laugh and the world laughs! The situation calls for an element of surprise, if not a well-pattered punch line. Work on your timing and delivery overnight. Focus on the buildup and on spitting out the words and swallowing the pauses at the right time. Then surprise us.

◀ ⏶ ⏷

Wonder reversed

W is for "Wonder." *Say the word!* The **W**-Rune reversed is about the power of laughter to cure what ails you. An artful play on words in the middle. . . an ironic twist at the end . . . a dose of satire . . . a dash of irony. Life itself is a comedy of manners (or is that errors?). To appreciate the joke, though, you may have to establish some distance. It looks like somebody needs some cheering up. So wipe that tear from your own eye first. And—for a moment at least—stop taking it all so seriously. Smile a little. *Traditional names: Wunjo reversed, The Joy. Generosity. Hospitality. Good Humor.*

For WORK questions. Come to the wiener roast! Whatever you did, it must have been amusing, because it looks like you're in for a ribbing now. Or else it's one of your business associates who has become the butt of the joke. It's all in good fun, mind you. But if some of these barbs stick, well then, you'll have to get out tweezers.

For LOVE questions. Return to laughter! Every relationship has its high points and low moments. But personally, I'd rather hear you giggling between the sheets than cutting each other down. It's time to create one of those moments that not only sustains you but reminds you why you got together in the first place.

For MONEY questions. Funny money! It's nothing to laugh at, I'm sure. But you have to admit all this accounting magic and creative financing is pretty funny. The out-years may look great, but all in all the numbers are a crock. Well, you can't blame them for trying.

For STRATEGY questions. Humor them! The situation is more than ironic, it's ridiculous—even ludicrous in its way. And you can't help but laugh at how silly it all looks when you see it from a couple of paces back. Why wait to look back on it all later and laugh? Go ahead, laugh now.

H Ⓗ

Hail

H is for "Hail" *Say the word!* The **H**-Rune is about the powers of nature . . . to shape and mold the world . . . to change the environment . . . and help or hinder your safe passage. A storm must be kicking up in your neck of the woods. And I'd have to say all hail's about to break loose. Why else would a dark cloud be hovering over your head? Perhaps you'd best come in, before you catch a cold. The best you can do sometimes is weather these things. You need to ride out this storm. Batten down the hatches for now. Put tape on the windows. Make popcorn, and get out the hurricane lamps. Tomorrow is soon enough to pick up the pieces. *Traditional names: Hagalaz, The Hail. The Hailstone. White Stone of the Frost Giant. The Hail Egg.*

For WORK questions. Fallout attack! The rumblings from the executive tower are growing noticeably louder. And the grapevine is going rat-a-tat-tat. But as tragic as the buzz may make it out to be, it will most certainly result in new opportunities for those willing to seize them.

For LOVE questions. Lovers' spat! Now, now, I don't know who did what first—or to whom—but the claws and fangs are a bit much. If you must quarrel, at least tape your hands and put on boxing gloves. Into your corners, guys. Now that verbal punches have been thrown, it's time to kiss and make up, isn't it? (And it's the best part.)

For MONEY questions. Hazard insurance! You can't possibly guard against every contingency. But it never hurts to review the insurance coverage you're carrying . . . or the premiums you're paying for peace of mind. Shop around. Try to get the best deal. (And don't let them prey on your healthy fear.)

For STRATEGY questions. Seek cover! This situation is probably not as dangerous as it appears—though it looks pretty dark and ominous out there right now. It might be a good idea to get out that old security blanket of yours and snuggle up with your thumb and your toes for a while. If the storm gets too scary, you can always hightail it to the basement. (But yikes! Who wants to go down there?)

✝ Ⓝ

Need

N is for "Need." *Say the word!* The **N**-Rune is about the power of the human will to survive . . . despite the fiercest conditions and against the world's worst odds. At this time, you are in want of something so badly that it is like a hunger or a thirst. The need burns away at your insides, and no matter what you do, it keeps coming back. It's possible you are down on your luck, up to your eyebrows, or in over your waist. If so, I know you can make it, for these days are numbered just like all the rest. Take them as they come, and don't let them color your attitude wrong. It's not all over till it's done. And I can see you're hanging in there with a vengeance to the bitter end. *Traditional names: Naudhiz, The Need. Necessity. The Need-Fire. A Fire Struck by Steel, Flint, and Tinder.*

For WORK questions. Pecking order! It's a competitive place, all right. And we all have our needs for status and prestige. Some even get a good parking space. (But it's anything but free!) Don't let the lesser get the better of you. Rise to your highest level of confidence.

For LOVE questions. Not tonight! I guess you might say the two of you have different needs. Or maybe it's simply that one of you can't keep up with the other. Unfortunately, in this discussion there's no way to win for losing. Someone's bound to feel guilty, used, or hurt. Oh, well. Might as well call it a night.

For MONEY questions. Cash shortfall! Something comes up missing at the end of the day. You wind up short-changed, short-sheeted, or even short-sticked. What's gone's gone, I guess. What's done's done. It looks like you'll have to run a little in the red. But by cutting costs, you'll recover your losses in time. (Besides, you can probably take a write-off.)

For STRATEGY questions. Prioritize! The situation requires you to do without a little something—at least for a while. All in all, you have no choice but to make the sacrifice. Yet you have many choices among the things you could give up. Pick something that you won't really miss all that much.

I Ⓞ

Ice

I is for "Ice." *Say the word!* The **I**-Rune is about the power of cold to freeze and heat to melt. One way hardens, and the other liquefies. Perhaps you're running hot or cold yourself. Or is it that you're feeling lukewarm about it? But I don't think so—this passion runs too deep to be tepid. And this kind of trouble is usually either very thick or wafer-thin. What is it you need to lock away so carefully? What are you trying to hold on to? Or hold in? Whatever this secret is, it needs to be kept on ice until you figure out what to do about it. Or else, something needs to be frozen in its tracks. If someone's been giving you a hard time, nip it in the bud right now. Put a stop to unwelcome advances. By closing this up, you open the way. *Traditional names: Isa, The Ice. Ice on the River. The Temporary Road.*

For WORK questions. Hockey puck! The boundaries are pretty much frozen. The organizational chart is burnt onto the drum of the photocopier. And all the titles are chiseled in brass. Once again the pieces on the board are placed . . . knight, bishop, and rook to the rear, and all the pawns on the front line. Is this a game of wits or what? Use yours.

For LOVE questions. Silver skates! It was a glittering night. The trees were full of twinkle lights—or was it really icicles reflecting the moonlight? There were certainly stars in your eyes . . . and not a moment's hesitation. How could one moment change everything so permanently? You're committed now . . . trapped? . . . or is it released?

For MONEY questions. Cash poor! It's all tied up in tax-deferred annuities, land, or automobiles. And even if there aren't substantial penalties for early withdrawal, there are significant delays in getting a payout. You're up a creek without your gold card. So your assets are frozen for a while—at least they're assets.

For STRATEGY questions. Lock in your votes! The situation is firming up quickly. So you must jockey for position and then stay put. Nobody is going to be going anyplace fast for a while. Nothing that isn't already scheduled is going to get done. Everything settles down into suspended animation. So you should have plenty of time to plot your next moves.

◇ Ⓨ ⒜ Ⓙ ⒡

Year

Y is for "Year." *Say the word!* The **Y**-Rune is about the power of time. So either you have an old wound to heal, my friend, or else you've got a long-term plan to realize. Either way, time is the answer. The great year runs its perpetual cycle through, from solstice to solstice . . . from equinox to equinox . . . till 12-odd moons have waxed and waned the nights away. You note the dates and times of your appointments. You watch the clock. The hours, days, weeks, and years themselves add up. You too cycle through your nights and days. What you start today gets done tomorrow. And everything comes back around. *Traditional names: Jera, The Year. The Harvest Time. Spring and Fall. The Fruitful Year. The Cycle of Change.*

For WORK questions. Give it a year! There are some definite possibilities here. But what they will amount to in the long run, nobody knows for sure. You need to get through the whole cycle before it will be clear. Twelve months from now you will be in a much better position to judge what it is worth to you . . . and why.

For LOVE questions. September love! There's a harvest moon up in the sky . . . and shine on, shine on, the two of you. The scent of burning leaves and frying food is on the air. And the breeze is down from Canada. It makes you wish you had a fireplace or some wood to burn in it. But mostly you have this incredible urge to nest. Stock up for the winter.

For MONEY questions. Compounded annual yield! These are only projections, of course. But based on historic averages—and no one can predict what the market will do—you should see a two-digit return on your investment over time. All well and good. Though nothing is certain, it's always good to think ahead.

For STRATEGY questions. Plan for the future! The situation you are in requires you to project your results forward. Where is it you want to be 365 days from now? And just how are you going to get there from here? In the process of deciding what to do when, take advantage of cyclical events and factor in seasonalities. To get by, you may need to borrow in one season to pay back in another. So be it.

↓ Ê Ǝ

hElp

Ê is for "hElp." *Say the word!* The Ê-Rune is about the power of endurance. But is it stamina or fortitude that gets you through? A physical ailment makes you feel weak in the knees or weary in the head. Did you do something to bring this pain upon yourself? Or was it the behavior of others that victimized you? What are the symptoms, signs, and omens? What do you do that aggravates your condition? If no real illness afflicts you, then I guess you are simply worried that one may . . . someday. It is time, my friend, to revitalize your poor old bones and soothe your troubled head. This is the Rune that guarded the souls of the dead. It signals good health, long life, and the strength to endure old age. *Traditional names: Eihwaz, The Yew. A Yew Tree. The Evergreen. The Bow of Yew.*

For WORK questions. Occupational hazard! Looks like tennis elbow to me. Or did pushing all that paper for a living give you a nasty cut on your finger? Well, don't ask me, I'm not the doc. And if you want to find an attorney, you'll have to turn on the TV. But I'll tell you this: Living has its price. And you can't blame everything on everyone else.

For LOVE questions. Sexually transmitted! You can't get it from kissing or holding hands . . . from toilet seats or swimming pools . . . or even from smoking cigarettes together. Well, as the pope and surgeon general concur, you can always abstain. Don't do anything I shouldn't, my friend.

For MONEY questions. Health insurance! At these rates, who can afford to be well, let alone sick? I guess all that medical technology costs a pretty penny, huh? Pay the premiums they demand, or else run the risk of not having a bedpan to sit in. Turn your head and cough, my friend.

For STRATEGY questions. Quality of life! You're in a situation in which you can only call some of the shots. Life itself is a risk. And it's not possible to get the odds down to zero. I fear you are going to worry yourself silly. Try to put these things into perspective.

ᚴ ⓟ

hoPe

P is for "hoPe." *Say the word!* The **P**-Rune is about the power of the Runes themselves . . . to guide and direct you . . . to help you achieve your goals . . . to even bring you luck. It looks like you've been grasping at straws lately. Or else you've been high-rolling the dice. You know, you are free to wish for <u>whatever</u> you want—at least around these parts. But you and I both know, it is your own actions that usually influence the outcome—and not just luck. It's all pretty much a question of how badly you want your wish . . . and how long you're willing to work and wait to get it. You might want to plot a few short-term goals as intermediate targets. *Traditional names: Perthro, The Dice Cup. Runes Made from an Apple Tree. A Game of Chance.*

For WORK questions. Three-year forecast! Out there on your strategic planning horizon, there sits a vision statement. So this is where you think you're going, huh? This is where you think you'll be? I don't know, it looks pretty ambitious. But if you get into a pinch, you can always restructure.

For LOVE questions. Check the personals! But you better brush up on your mating terms first. I'd hate to see you wind up with an SM/BD in BVDs . . . who smokes (unless, of course, that's what you're in the market for). Well, it never hurts to advertise. Just remember there's such a thing as being too specialized. True love doesn't need a scorecard.

For MONEY questions. Lucky penny! It would, of course, be illegal and practically sacrilegious to bore a hole through this perfectly good copper relief of Honest Abe's face. But wasn't it the Father of our Country who made a wish on a silver dollar? And look what it did for him! Heck, it's not good for anything but making change anyway. You might as well put it in your pocket for luck, my friend.

For STRATEGY questions. Take your pick! You're in a situation in which you can choose any prize on the top row . . . just as soon as you knock over these raggedy dolls. Three balls for a buck, pal. So what do you say? You game? Or are you just gonna watch? If somebody's gotta win, it might as well be a big spender like you.

⤨ ⓙ

hoPe reversed

P is for "ho**P**e." *Say the word!* The **P**-Rune reversed is about the power of the Runes themselves . . . to help you respond to negative situations . . . to counteract destructive influences . . . and to stand off temptations. Strange as it may seem, someone does not wish you well in your endeavors right now. Maybe you have inadvertently intimidated them. Or perhaps they just don't understand. Sure, it would be nice to have everyone's enthusiastic backing and support. But if you hope to achieve your dream, you can't help but worry a few individuals—or even threaten some—in the process of making your breakthrough. Let them nay-say. But don't let their negative energy get to you. Wipe the dust from your shoes. And go your separate way. *Traditional names: Perthro, The Dice Cup. The Poisoned Apple*.

For WORK questions. One bad apple! Something's rotten in the state of Denmark (or is that D.C.?) And you'd better flesh it out pretty fast, because it's starting to smell like a barnyard in here. But no matter how much it would appear to be one person's problem, you know, of course, that everyone's a little to blame.

For LOVE questions. Could I tempt you! Well, an apple a day, they say . . . and all work and no play. These fruits are almost too delectable to resist—maybe even too good to be true. If God didn't mean for you to have it, why would She have put it in the center of your Universe? Still, you'd best think about it once more before you listen to the serpent.

For MONEY questions. Venture capital! This is a long shot if ever there was one, my friend. And the return—if any—is speculative. Many things stand in the way. And as many more will have to go right in order to turn a profit. You are free to put up the money if you'd like to play for the big stakes—but you may have to go for broke in the process. Negotiate an escape clause.

For STRATEGY questions. Be forewarned! You're in a situation in which the motives of others are not obvious or necessarily pure. Something that looks like an opportunity may be a roadblock in disguise—and vice versa. The dreams and aspirations of others clash with yours, but in most cases there is sufficient overlap to strike a compromise.

Ψ ☒

reSIStance

Z is for "reSIStance." *Say the word!* The **Z**-Rune is about the power to ward things off . . . manipulative people, dangerous ideas, and anything else that threatens your mental condition, physical state, or spiritual well-being. This is the Rune that keeps danger out . . . and locks what needs to be protected in. Having drawn the **Z**-Rune, it looks like you're in need of some protection right now. But is it something outside that threatens you? Or is it something on the inside that is trying to get at you? It wouldn't hurt to cover both ends, I guess. But all in all, there's no need to worry. You're going to come through everything okay—the **Z**-Rune practically guarantees it. *Traditional names: Elhaz, The Elk. The Antlers of an Elk. The Falcon's Claw. The Raised Hand of Protection.*

For WORK questions. Flexible leave! Looks to me like you're due for a few mental health days all in a row. Perhaps a long weekend is what the doctor ordered. Or how about taking a floating holiday in the middle of the week? And if no national or religious holiday is in sight, you can always hold out hope for a snow day. If all else fails, take a long lunch.

For LOVE questions. Hermetically sealed! And speaking of nooners . . . I know that at certain moments nothing else matters. But one thing never changes: You can alter your whole destiny in ten minutes or less. Lovers' feelings are hurt routinely in the process. Some even pine away from making love (especially these days). You can't go through life sealed in plastic. But if I were you, I'd at least keep my Runes covered.

For MONEY questions. Overdraft protection! Been writing a lot of checks lately? Lucky you've got that line-o-credit to back them up. Well, you gotta eat, and roughage isn't getting any cheaper. You may have to pay interest on the outstanding balance of your loans, but at least you can avoid the penalties and processing fees for returned checks.

For STRATEGY questions. Every man for herself! You're in a situation in which—regardless of your age, race, color, creed, gender, and sexual preference (or smoking, drinking, height, or weight status)—you need to get by as best you can. There are those who will discriminate against you on nothing more than the color of your eyes or the cut of your jeans (or is that genes?). Lucky you're protected by the Constitution. But just in case, stick up for your rights, enumerated or not.

✈ Ⓩ

reSIStance reversed

Z is for "reSIStance." *Say the word!* The **Z**-Rune reversed is about the power to make peace . . . both with each other and yourself. I don't know what kind of holy war you were on (or was it a vendetta?). And I'm not sure whether the enemy was real, or just a figment of your vivid imagination. But I do know this: It's time to end the fighting and bring the troops back home now. Call for a summit. Sit down at the bargaining table. Draw some new lines on the paper, and agree to the terms and conditions of the settlement. Then tear down the barricades. Shut down the propaganda machine. Put your weapons, your bile, and your vitriol away. Shake hands. And resolve to never, ever do this to yourself again. *Traditional names: Elhaz, The Elk. The Elk Sedge. The Marsh Grasses.*

For WORK questions. Bury the hatchet! . . . and preferably not in somebody else's back this time. Enough's enough already. This little game has gone about as far as it really ought to go. If one has to make the first concession, it might as well be you. I guess you can figure out for yourself how to do it and still save face.

For LOVE questions. Joint agreement! It's nice to see the two of you on speaking terms. It's a good sign that everything can be worked out to your mutual satisfaction. Just keep talking and working at it. But it looks like everything's going to come out in the wash.

For MONEY questions. Amicable settlement! I'm afraid you're going to have to pay back the money you owe before you can be done with this. Why not settle out of court and save yourself the legal fees? Set up a reasonable payment plan, and get on with the rest of your life.

For STRATEGY questions. Amenable terms! The situation you are in demands that you pass the peace pipe. (But you don't have to really smoke it, if it's against your religion.) The point is, you need to reach agreement with each other, in terms that you can both live with—at least for the foreseeable future. Work it out.

Ƨ Ⓢ

Sun & Stars

S is for "Sun." **S** is for "Stars." *Say the words!* The **S**-Rune is about the power to follow your star, set your sights, find your direction, and lock in on your own course. You must be feeling rather disoriented. Or else, for the first time, you aren't wondering anymore. The sun, moon, and stars are fixed in the sky—it seems—for many reasons, one of which is to point the way. Your Runes can do the same, but I'll let you be the judge of them. If I were you, though, I'd take this one as a sign that the end of your travail is near. Perhaps the truth was just too blinding—or too obvious—to see at first. But now that you've put on your polarized shades, it's practically glare-free. For once, you can see everything clearly, including the path stretched out in front of you. *Traditional names: Sowilo, The Sun. The Sun Wheel. Lightning. The Sun Shield.*

For WORK questions. Due north! Let's see now. Just follow the Pointer Stars in the bowl of the Big Dipper . . . over to the tail of the Little Dipper . . . and that little faint one right yonder is the North Star. Head that way. Or I guess you could use a compass, but wouldn't it kind of take the sport out of it? At any rate, you'll soon be getting new marching orders. Even so, your destiny is only partially determined for you.

For LOVE questions. Star-Crossed Lovers! What light through yonder window breaks? Is it just the east, Romeo? Or is someone signaling you? How can the dawn come so soon, or the evening fly so quickly? Do not fear. This is the nightingale you hear . . . and not the lark. Hold on to the night.

For MONEY questions. Western Union! Transfer funds now. Stop. Buy low. Sell high. Stop. An opportunity like this comes along once in a blue moon. Stop. But . . . I wouldn't stop now if I were you. Make hay while the sun shines.

For STRATEGY questions. The Southern Cross! You're in a situation right now that is already giving you plenty of clues on its own. But sometimes the most obvious things are the most difficult to unravel. Trust your own eyes, ears, and nose. The writing is on the wall. And it's as clear as the Rune in your fist.

↑ Ⓣ

Triumph

T is for "Triumph." *Say the word!* The **T**-Rune is about the power of politics . . . to mobilize the masses, generate support from the grass roots, and achieve political consensus. I see you participating in a public works project of some kind, going to a meeting, or attending a rally. Whatever your favorite cause, your patriotic spirit is out there waving the flag. Your school spirit is doing a cheer. And your team spirit is bringing up the rear. You might even be on the front line of a popular movement or the cutting edge of a new technology. And if you can't be in the forefront, do what you can from home. Put up posters. Plant placards in yards. Make calls. And if you've got any of that yellow ribbon left, there're plenty more trees on down the street. Others want to get you on their side. Back a winner. *Traditional names: Tiwaz—The Warrior. Tyr—The God of War. Tiw—The Noble Hero. Patron of Tuesday.*

For WORK questions. PR campaigns! Someone's making flower arrangements of the truth . . . or at least one version of it. Balloons are being blown up. Slogans are being crafted. Speeches, memos, and public statements are being prepared for release. It looks like someone's either bucking for a promotion . . . or trying to hang on to a job. Victory comes to the one who is most convincing.

For LOVE questions. March on Washington! Something about your lifestyle seems to be at odds with the laws on the books. Public sentiment in general is mixed. And no politician wants to touch your cause in an election year. Yet perhaps there is enough strength in your numbers to make a convincing argument. Lucky you have the right to peaceably assemble. But don't forget to get a permit in advance.

For MONEY questions. The market rallies! News of lowering interest rates—or some other government action—brings investor confidence back. At least for the moment, the market is bullish. But you will have to act fast to take advantage of this upswing. Invest in the industries that should benefit most from the rumors of war or the prospect of possible settlement.

For STRATEGY questions. Stand up and be counted! The situation you are in requires you to step forward, enlist, or volunteer for active duty. And you might as well go along willingly, because if you don't, they have ways of making you fall in line. Destructive forces are at work. You might as well seize the opportunity. If you act fast enough and fight hard enough, you might even get a medal.

↓ ①

Triumph reversed

T is for "Triumph." *Say the word!* The **T**-Rune reversed is about the power of politics . . . to pull the wool over your eyes, to divert attention from the real issues, and to back you into a corner. Things are not exactly what they seem. People are saying one thing, doing another, and hoping that they won't get caught before it's too late to stop the wheels already in motion. All their arguments are tied with striped bows and star-spangled bunting. Their reasons smell like hot apple pie with cinnamon. They can look you straight in the eye and tell a lie. A fool is born every seventeen seconds—don't you be one of them. Carry the **T**-Rune in your pocket to triumph over the political bull-geois. *Traditional names: Tiwaz reversed, The Warrior. The Sky God. God of Moral Judgment. Keeper of Oaths.*

For **WORK** *questions.* Hardball! It's in your court now. But it would have been nice had they waited for you to get your racket out and your shoes tied. The possibility of being blindsided, rearended, or upstaged is relatively high right now. And if I were you, I wouldn't turn my back, let alone bend over.

For **LOVE** *questions.* Skeletons in the attic! If you have anything you'd like to keep hidden, you'd better cover your tracks well, my friend. This is not, after all, a jury of your peers. And your enemies would embarrass you in public if it meant another vote for their side. Some would even sell you out if the price were right. So beware. But mostly, be selective in choosing your bedfellows . . . especially the stranger ones.

For **MONEY** *questions.* Such a deal! It's nice to have the use of this money. But what kinds of strings are attached? Who are you beholden to? And incidentally, what's the interest rate? I advise you to get it all in writing up front. And be sure to read the fine print before you initial it here . . . here . . . and on the back. The best swindlers are politicians in disguise.

For **STRATEGY** *questions.* Power politics! The situation you are in is not what it seems. Someone is feeding you a plate of red herring or telling you half a truth. The question is, do you really trust this person? Or is that slick exterior a dead giveaway itself? Destructive forces are still at work. This is one of those opportunities you might want to pass up.

Birth

B is for "Birth." *Say the word!* The **B**-Rune is about the power of the creative process . . . to give form, shape, and substance to things . . . to breathe new life into a tired old soul . . . to even bring new life itself into being. This is a creative, productive, and fertile time. It is as if spring has come overnight. The forsythia is blooming golden, and everything else is greening up. You are virtually blossoming yourself. What a healthy specimen you have become in your newfound youth. Keep making your music. Keep dancing your dance. (And I don't care which ear you want to pierce.) It's also possible, of course, that someone in your life is actually pregnant. If the signs are not obvious to you by now, you'll see for yourself soon enough. Just in case, congratulations. *Traditional names: Berkano, The Birches. The First Tree to Green. The Bringer of Fertility.*

For **WORK** *questions.* Return to normalcy! Wow! With productivity like this, we'll have to expand to another place. I knew it was only a temporary downturn . . . just a momentary lapse in enthusiasm. But boy-oh-boy! It's good to be back, isn't it? And you still have it, don't you? It's all in the palm of your hand. You can do no wrong.

For **LOVE** *questions.* Makin' babies! Well, it's that time of the month. There's a great big Egg Moon in the sky. And the lady's temperature is rising. I'd hate for you to feel under any pressure about it, but the night's not getting any younger . . . and neither are we. Just remember there are already six billion of us—and we're almost out of parking spaces. (Ah, but what do I know?) Give us a genius.

For **MONEY** *questions.* Early maturation! Whatever deal this is, it's about to pay off on an accelerated schedule. Even discounting for inflation, the rate of return is better than money in the bank. And then, of course, there is the tax advantage. Heck, you must have a green thumb—or is it a money tree?

For STRATEGY questions. Be prolific! The situation you are in calls for you to form many buds, bear many blossoms, spread lots of pollen . . . and harvest as much fruit as you can. Everything is progressing at its normal rate—at least the normal rate for you. Just go at your own pace. And don't be discouraged if your efforts are not the first to be rewarded. Some that bloom late bear the better fruit.

◣ ⑨

Birth reversed

B is for "re**B**irth." *Say the word!* The **B**-Rune reversed is about the power to start all over again. The feeling you are experiencing is like an itch that periodically needs to be scratched. And this must be the seventh year, my friend, because the itch is back. You are about to come out of your shell, shed your skin, and be reborn . . . again. That old, familiar feeling is back. And it's a dead giveaway. But it doesn't mean you have to repeat yourself. How will you play your hand this time? How will you rearrange your life? And what will you do for an encore? Every transition has its turning point. Carry the **B**-Rune to ease you through your upcoming rite of passage. *Traditional names: Berkano reversed, The Birches. The Switch Made of Birch.*

For WORK questions. One rung at a time! And no pushing! It looks like you've filled out the same forms—or drunk the same company coffee—long enough. You'd like to move on to something else that's a bit more challenging. Or maybe you'd be happy with a simple change of pace. Apply for an internal opening. Or else, type up your resumé and get it in the mail.

For LOVE questions. Midlife crisis! Love is always sweeter the second time around—well, so they say. But is there something you missed out on the first time? Or is it just that you know now what you wish you'd known then? I'd give you a friendly word of advice, but you'll probably go ahead with it anyway. One way or the other, you will make your transition.

For MONEY questions. Stock portfolio! It's time to review your investment strategy. Add up the money you've amassed on paper. Calculate the respective rates of return. Devise new schemes for leveraging your assets and putting your money to work for you. Plan far enough in advance for retirement, and maybe you can even take it early.

For STRATEGY questions. Revitalization! You are in a situation that demands a spring cleaning, a fresh coat of paint, or a whole new look. One way to look young is to act young. One way to act young is to feel young. And one way to feel young is to do something rash and impetuous. How about pursuing that old dream of yours? Or else we could show each other our tattoos.

M ⓔ

fEmale

E is for "fEmale." *Say the word!* The **E**-Rune is about the power of women's intuition . . . to know things without having any way of knowing them and to be able to pick up on things in advance. You can read the signs for yourself, and you've been getting plenty of clues to choose from lately. An odd fragment of a dream lingers with you through the day. A random thought flashes through your head, ringing with the truth. Gazing into space, you see a vision. And you can't keep your hands off your Runes. How could you be imagining these things? If you think so-and-so might drop by, you clean. If you think what's-his-name might phone, you are not surprised when your Call Waiting button beeps. It's the same little coincidences over and over again that create your larger body of evidence. If you take the trouble to see them, you will never want for the signs. *Traditional names: Ehwaz, The Horse. The Sacred White Horse. The Chariot of the Sun. The Messenger of the Gods.*

For WORK questions. Burning ears! Yes. If you think someone's talking about you behind your back, you're absolutely correct. In fact, the whole workplace is probably buzzing about it by now. Ah, what the heck? Let 'em say what they will. What do they know?

For LOVE questions. Shivers up the spine! One thing's for sure: Somebody just had a good time around here. (Either that, or who just walked on my grave?) And speaking of sex and death, you know they say that there's a fine line, my friend, between pleasure and pain. You know what you know, I guess. You feel what you feel—and you don't feel what you don't feel. Go with your instincts.

For **MONEY** *questions.* Itchy palms! Yes, indeed, my friend. You're soaking in dishwashing liquid. And those nails of yours are soon to be polished with silver. Cross my palm, and I'll tell you more. Only $3.95 a minute. (Just kidding.) Draw another Rune— it's on the house. And wait for the check that's surely in the mail.

For **STRATEGY** *questions.* Intuit your way! You're in a situation that reveals itself to you in mysterious ways. All you really have to do is be attentive for the signs. But mind you, some of them will be false alarms, and the only way to know for sure is to know for yourself. The truth always feels deep, dark, and calm when it comes. Accept no substitutes.

ꠝꠛ

fEmale reversed

E is for "fEmale." *Say the word!* The **E**-Rune reversed is about the power of a man's gut feelings . . . to pick up on subtle clues, to sense danger, and to heed a welcome warning. You don't need to see any more numbers on this one, pal. There's hardly any dog and pony show or song and dance that could change your position now. It's something you can't really put your finger on. Maybe it was a shifty look in the eyes. Or perhaps the handshake was too weak or too brief. I don't know. (And neither do you.) Though other parts of your anatomy may be saying yes, yes, your gut is telling you no, no, no. I'd go with these female feelings, if I were you. And if you don't believe me, then put two and two together for yourself. *Traditional names: Ehwaz reversed, The Horse. The White Horse on the Hill. The White Stallion. The Steed of Odin.*

For **WORK** *questions.* Horse chute! Either you're riding bucking broncs for a living, or else it's getting pretty deep in here for less conspicuous reasons. Well, when the manure's been spread this heavy, you can smell it from three miles off. Get out your handkerchief and cover your nose if you must. Steer clear of the road apples.

For **LOVE** *questions.* Hung like a horse! Built like a brick outhouse? Well now, isn't this the American dream come true? Or was that a Russian legend? I must confess I'm not exactly sure how to touch this one, except with a very long stick. I'd keep a little more distance if I were you. (But then again, I'm not.)

For MONEY questions. Day at the races! They're at the post. The gates are down, and . . . they're off and running. (Come on, Moe-Joe.) And it's neck and neck at the backstretch . . . by a nose at the turn . . . and coming up on the outside . . . (Yes!) It's Moe-Joe by an eighth. I guess you had a lucky hunch? What did it pay?

For STRATEGY questions. Go with your gut! You're in a situation not unlike any other, except that for some reason you have this funny inkling about this one . . . and it's not necessarily good. Something's gnawing at your innards. Or is it gripping at your outards? You know better by now not to ignore these signals . . . don't you? Take a timely tip from your taut gut.

ᛗ Ⓜ

Male

M is for "Male." *Say the word!* The **M**-Rune is about the power of reason, intelligence, and rational thought . . . to change both the world around you and the world itself. So go right ahead. But first you might want to check the printouts and data tables. Mathematical facts, scientific data, and empirical evidence are involved. To find your answer, first consult your charts and graphs. But human logic also plays its part. You will have to draw the conclusions for yourself. Put your mind to work on it. Focus. Concentrate. Search your memory for prior art. Check all the computations for accuracy. Hunt up the right words. Then announce your conclusions to the world. One way to achieve the things you want is to do them by the book. *Traditional names: Mannaz, The Man. Humankind. Descendants of the Gods. The Wise Man.*

For WORK questions. Think tank! What is it you do in there all day? Are you searching for the cure to cancer? Or is it just another one of your moneymaking schemes? What new electrical appliance are you going to give us next? And will we be able to set the clock on it this time? Go with the latest consumer research. But sometimes the public doesn't predict itself very well. Keep tinkering with that elusive idea.

For LOVE questions. Pros and cons! This is a tough one to call. You are inclined to want to list the good points on one side of the paper and the bad points on the other. Then weigh, check, and balance to see if you can get the whole thing to break even or wash clean. It's not the best way to make this decision, but you have to go with your strengths. Look at all the numbers, but in the end, listen to your heart.

For MONEY questions. Dollars and cents! The net result is as clear as the ink that's not even dry on the page. Read it for yourself. It's all there in black and white—with maybe a drop or two of red. (Is that your blood?) Well, you win some, you lose some. Now, where do we go from here?

For STRATEGY questions. Analyze it to death! The situation you are in requires you to assume a detached distance and an objective point of view. The important thing to do first is gather the facts. But sooner or later you're going to have to synthesize the data into a conclusion—and that takes an intuitive leap. Sleep on it, and note how you "feel" in the morning. (But if I were you, I wouldn't tell anyone I got this advice from my Runes.)

ᛗ ⓦ

Male reversed

M is for "Male." *Say the word!* The **M**-Rune reversed is about the power of mere mortals to figure things out on their own. In your efforts to understand things, you have created many similes, metaphors, and fairy tales. And there seems to be a moral to every story. Your condition is much like other things in the world. It should be easy to see the similarity between what's happening in your life and what's happened elsewhere before. But it is mostly a matter of proportion, scale, and viewpoint. You may need to get outside yourself in order to get a clearer view. Or someone else may be willing to draw a few analogies for you. Something theoretical or philosophical is involved. (Is this a Rune, Plato—or just an example of one?) *Traditional names: Mannaz reversed, The Man. Mere Mortals. The Man in the Moon. The Measurer of Time. The Wise Woman.*

For WORK questions. The corporate myth! In the beginning was the Founding Father's dream. On nothing more than a couple of bucks and a pocketful of ambition, this little endeavor was built into a thriving enterprise. But he never could have done it without you. (And how could he forget it?) I see a coffee mug or a besloganed T-shirt in your future. Wear it in good health.

For LOVE questions. A fairy-tale ending! Once upon a time, there were these two young kids who didn't know any better. They thought they were in love! So they got married and had kids (not necessarily in that order). They pinched a few dollars and built a little life for themselves. And damn, if they didn't live practically ever after.

For MONEY questions. This little piggy! Why do I smell roast beef, mashed potatoes, and gravy? And was that you going wee-wee, wee-wee? The moral of the story is glad but true. Some get taken to market. Some stay home in bed. But you get to count your money all the way to the automatic teller.

For STRATEGY questions. Just like in the movies! The situation you are in is vaguely reminiscent of a show you saw once. Let's see now—who starred in it? What was the plot? And how did they so artfully resolve it? Would that life were like a screenplay. All you'd have to do is flip ahead to see how it all turns out—at least before the final cut. Write your own ending to this one.

ᚱ ᛚ

Love

L is for "Love." *Say the word!* The L-Rune is about the power of emotional tides . . . to bring you up and drag you under . . . to make you hate and cause you to love . . . and all in all to carry you along for the ride. That old pulse of yours is thump-thump-thumping, my friend. And is that your blood pressure I see on the rise? Something's got you mighty riled, all right. Or is it hot in here? If you want to slip into something more comfortable, I'll hold the place. You can at least loosen your collar, if not your vest. Or maybe a cold shower would put things in proper perspective. But seriously, you'll need friends as well as lovers to get through all the long nights. And if you want to talk it over with somebody, try a buddy or a trusted family member. *Traditional names: Laguz, The*

Water. The Sea. The River. The Power of Waves. The Moon and the Tides.

For WORK questions. A fish in water! It may not be the perfect home for you, but you take to it nonetheless. Soon you know your way around the place. And there's a certain comfort in charting where the shallow waters lie, as well as the treacherous depths. I guess you could say you've gotten your feet wet. At least you know who your friends are.

For LOVE questions. Swim the widest ocean! I guess there is no better way to describe how you feel than to measure it in terms of the lengths to which you would go. Well, my friend, I have nothing else to say but climb every mountain . . . ford every stream . . . drive every interstate. This one's good for as long as the mighty Mississip has a drop of water left in it.

For MONEY questions. Hook, line, and sinker! Looks like somebody's taken the bait. Well, what are you going to do when they look at you with those big baby blues? A friend, relative, or family member wants to borrow funds from you, sell you something, cut you in on the deal, or get you to pick up the tab. What's this friendship worth to you? I guess we'll soon find out now, won't we? Or could it be that a richer relative soon backs you?

For STRATEGY questions. Swim the extra mile! The situation you're in requires you to go the distance. So name your stroke, and I'll race you to the end of the pool. Of course, you can also tread water if you like. Or else float on your back. And if you feel yourself sinking, raise your hand and wave. If there's no lifeguard on duty, your friends will surely come to save you.

◀ ⑦

Love reversed

L is for "Love." *Say the word!* The L-Rune reversed is about the power of unseen currents to pull you in directions you did not necessarily wish to go. The situation is on the verge of being out of control. Something is getting away from you . . . or has already escaped your notice. And it's the craziest thing how something that looks so placid on the surface could yet be tumultuous underneath. Perhaps it's just a case of the opening-night jitters—and maybe I'm making a big deal out of nothing. A little stress and tension can give you a creative edge. But you might want to guard against mood swings at a time like this. *Traditional names: Laguz reversed, The Water. The Underworld. The Undercurrent. Black Realm of the Unknown. Moon Madness.*

For WORK questions. Troubled waters! Well, this is certainly not the River Kwai, but a big bridge needs to be built over this obstacle course. And it's going to have to be a team project. You'll need to lend a hand, even if you have mixed emotions about the goal.

For LOVE questions. Chill out! Are these the words of love I hear? Or is one of you just under a lot of pressure? or having a bad day? Hand me a tissue, will you? Let's dry your eyes. I know these words didn't mean what they said verbatim. It was all just a misunderstanding.

For MONEY questions. Try to stay calm! I think this venture has gone just about as far as it can without an infusion of capital. What you've sunk into it already is long down the drain. And it might be time to pull the plug on this one. Write off as much as you can as goodwill. And see if you can sell off the assets to somebody else.

For STRATEGY questions. Beware the moon! The situation you are in is not entirely your own doing. Forces outside your control are at work. Or powers outside your command are at play. You may need to run up a white flag, set off a flare, or even dial 911 (but only in an emergency). More likely you just need to get to the bottom of something. Once you understand the total situation, you will be in a better position to act.

✵ ⊗

beING

-ING is for "be**ING**." *Say the word!* The **ING**-Rune is about the power of sexual energy . . . not only to create new life, mind you, but also to inspire the current one. For there is much to be gained from both abstinence and indulgence that has little to do with procreation. But why am I telling _you_ this? You're the one who drew the sex Rune. Why don't you tell me? And let's see if your ears turn red, too. But seriously, you have to make your own decisions about these kinds of things. If you're going to put your sexual energy into sex acts, the only person you really have to impress is your partner. But if you're going to channel it into your work, you'll reach a much larger audience. *Traditional names: Ing, The Fertility God. Consort of the Earth Mother. The God Who Has Left Us. Lord of the Dead.*

For WORK questions. Constructive outlet! Though you may feel tense—even frustrated sometimes—and bothered to the point of distraction, it's just nature's way of keeping you motivated. Direct your energies up, out, and into the task at hand. And whatever you do, keep your hands off your co-workers.

For LOVE questions. Simultaneous orgasm!!! It could happen! But you'll have to work at it. The keywords are *practice* and *patience*. Try to put yourself in the other person's (er . . .) shoes. This is one of those situations in which both stamina and endurance count. Better take your vitamins.

For MONEY questions. Wet dreams! Ah, the allure of cold, hard cash—and plenty of assets all in the right places. Oh, how interest can multiply like jackrabbits on a full moon. It's quite an appealing game plan. But be careful about obsession with the almighty buck. Ulysses S. Grant and Susan B. Anthony make for strange bedfellows, all right. And loneliness has little fair market value.

For STRATEGY questions. Manual dexterity! You're in a situation in which one thing is bound to lead to another. The trick is setting the chain reaction in motion. Though it's possible you could just do what comes naturally, you will probably have better success if you work on your technique. Practice on yourself. Rehearse in a magic mirror.

☖ Ⓞ

hOme

O is for "hOme." *Say the word!* The O-Rune is about the power of your family traditions to remind you of the people in your past to provide context and continuity. It is about the power of your people's ways to give life a meaningful order and make you homesick for the homeland. It is about the sanctity and privacy of your own four walls to give you shelter, haven, and refuge from the cold, cruel world. And it is about the people whom you have shared a roof with. But most of all, it is about the ones you love . . . and the ones who love you back. The answer that you seek now is to be found in the ways of your own people. Learn the lessons of your family's history. And think thrice before discarding what is quaint, old-fashioned, or corny. When in need, turn to family first. And when you need someone to talk to, phone home. *Traditional names: Othala, The Home. The Place of Your Birth. The Homestead. The Birthright.*

For WORK questions. Working from home! I don't need to tell you, nothing in the workplace is anything like it used to be. Yet, come to think of it, didn't we all used to work out of our homes? Looks like everything old comes back around. Good luck in your newfound family enterprise.

For LOVE questions. Honey, I'm home! This is going to be interesting now, isn't it? And just when you thought you were getting to know each other so well. I guess you'll just have to lay down a few ground rules. Ah, it's not so hard. Just be sure to give each other a little quality time . . . alone as well as together.

For MONEY questions. Home equity! You can still get a line of credit on that little nest egg you've built up on paper. But you'll have to read the tax regulations carefully before you deduct either the interest or the points. (For further details, get IRS Publication KETCH-22.) Don't spend your children's inheritance all in one place.

For STRATEGY questions. Show me the way to go home! You're in a situation that finds you longing for the comforts of home, family, and friends. And I'd say it's about time for a little get-together or at least a trip down memory lane. Do something nice for those at a distance. And never take for granted those in the next room.

❖ Ⓞ

hOme reversed

O is for "hOme." *Say the word!* The **O**-Rune reversed is about the power to build a new home . . . to set off on your own for the first time . . . to pick up the pieces following a storm . . . or to move away when the time has come to move on. It looks like it's time to spread your wings, my friend, and take the big leap, as it were. I'd say the old house is about to be sold, the condo title transferred, or the apartment rented to somebody else. In your hurry to get to your new place, don't forget to say good-bye to the house where it all happened for you once. What was here is all there'll ever be of it now. And as for the memories, they are locked in time and space. And nothing can be changed. You are forever young in this old place. *Traditional names: Othala reversed, The Home. The Land of Your Birth. The Homeland. Inheritance.*

For WORK questions. Bon voyage! Well, friend, it's been real. And whether it was good while it lasted or the job from living hell, it's all behind you now. Take the old Rolodex and the family photos from the desk. Delete your personal correspondence from the computer memory banks, erase your pending voice mail, take one last look back, and close the door.

For LOVE questions. Moving day! They'll be here any moment now. And the emotions floating around in your stomach will be lost to the dust and the confusion of the movers. There is a long checklist of things to be done. And there is no time to think that you are doing them now for the very last time. Focus today on where you're headed and not where you're coming from. There will be plenty of time to remember it later.

For MONEY questions. Pack it up! I don't care if you want to use a brown paper bag to make the transfer, but in this day and age there's no reason to get your hands filthy handling the lucre. A change in banking institutions looks to be in order. Or perhaps you're switching accountants, tax firms, or financial advisors. Good luck with your new business associates.

For STRATEGY questions. Move on! The situation you're in requires you to make a transition. A line is drawn in time. From this moment forward, it's up to somebody else to deal with the things that go wrong here. When your old house has been completely emptied of any reminder, take a last look and you will see it was not a home at all, but just a shell that the time has come to shed. Good riddance. Let's move on.

ᛗ ⑦ ⑦

Destiny

D is for "Destiny." *Say the word!* The **D**-Rune is about the power of time . . . to give life its structure, to create continuity, and to provide the context for things. As one day ends, another begins. And so you make your way through life, living moment to moment and one day to the next. There is a time to work and a time to play . . . a time to rise and a time to lie back down again. Somewhere in the process, what is meant to be gets done. But it is only at the end of the day that you can look back and see it all for what it is . . . so far. My friend, at this very moment, your destiny is out there in the future, just waiting for you to create it now. Sunrise, sunset, and morning star—what will you do tomorrow? *Traditional names: Dagaz, The Day. The Twilight. The Dusk and the Dawn. The Coming of a New Day.*

For WORK questions. Career batting average! It's day in, day out anyway, so you might as well make a game of it. Besides, the time goes faster when you're busy playing "Beat the Clock." Better yet, do something you adore. Though you may grow weary from lack of sleep, you will never grow tired of the effort. And you will never feel as if you gave your life to the company store.

For LOVE questions. Kismet! This relationship adds up to what it adds up to, nothing more and nothing less. Now that you've given it some time to play itself out, you can start to see what the pattern and the rhythm is. It's possible that the two of you could still break the habits you have established. But it's more likely that what you see at this point is what you will get in the future. Is that okay with you? If not, you know what to do.

For MONEY questions. Spending pattern! Somewhere there's a big computer that knows everything you've charged in the past three years, where you shopped, and how much you are inclined to spend on a single spree. Maybe it's time you reviewed your spending pattern yourself. Study your bank statements and review your credit history. And if it's a financial rut you see, start extricating yourself immediately.

For STRATEGY questions. Day by day! Night by night! The situation you are in is an unfolding one. For life is like an unraveling thread. And yet there are cycles and patterns and rhythms to the whole thing. Once you spot the recurring themes, behaviors, and trends, you will be in a good position to not only predict what is going to happen in your life, but to exert some control over it. Use what you know to influence your own destiny. And if you haven't spotted the pattern yet, keep looking.

0

weird

The Blank Rune is about the power of uncertainty. But is it fear of the unknown that stops you dead in your tracks? Or is it that there are just so many options to choose from, you can't decide? It's a world of possibilities out there. And there are plenty of opportunities for those who like a friendly game of hide-and-seek. Some chances even fall in your lap. But you've got to recognize them for what they are, even if they land upside down and backwards. The future is a blank book—intimidating and exhilarating at once. Out there somewhere, everything that's going to be is already written. All you have to do is take the pen in hand. This is your story, my friend. It belongs to you. And only you can write it . . . no matter how weird it turns out in the end. *Say the word. Traditional names: None, but it could stand for The Wyrd, A Person's Fate. That Which Is Written.*

For WORK questions. Stranger than fiction! The workplace has a tendency to seem like a three-ring circus or a carnival sideshow these days. And if you wrote down everything that happened, no one would ever believe it—I know. Yet companies and schools and governments seem to survive despite themselves . . . somehow. Even chaos has been known to resemble order. I guess this is one of those times.

For LOVE questions. Someone's out there! And he, she, or it is just waiting for you to come along. I know it sounds like complete and utter drivel. But I also know it's true. Everybody not only needs somebody, but there's a certain someone out there for everyone. So, though it may seem like a big void sometimes—or a crapshoot with incredible odds—everything is connected. Look for the meaning in every relationship.

For MONEY questions. Blank check! Well, my friend, it looks like you are free to write your own ticket. Or is that a line of credit? Your guess about how to invest it is as good as mine. There's no sure way to hedge the market, after all. And there's no telling what scheme will get rich quick next. In this volatile global economy, the best you can do is <u>attempt</u> to assure your own financial security. Plan ahead as best you can. And don't take anything for granted.

For STRATEGY questions. Weird science! The situation you are in demands that you take things into your own two hands. Believe what you will, but never that life is futile. With all these Runes at your disposal, how could you ever want for ammunition? Do what you will with them. But harm no one, not even in self-defense. Merry we have met, my friend. And merry we shall meet again.

Appendix

HOW TO GET YOUR MONEY'S WORTH
(*From* Runes in Ten Minutes)

There are basically three ways to use this book . . .

■ Open to Reading #1 and start playing along. If you take this route, you'll be guided through a series of question-and-answer sessions. The book will walk you through it. And the best part is, the only thing you have to learn is the answers to your own questions.

■ No Runes? No problem! If you don't have Runes or Scrabble® tiles yet, you can take a Runeless path through the book. Just start with Reading #4. The other Readings you can do without Runes are: #5, #6, #7, #10, #11, #12, #13, #20, #21, #22, and #23. This is also the path to take if you'd like the Runes to give you your personality profile.

■ You'd rather freestyle? Be my guest. Any time you're ready to fly solo, check out the notes in Reading #24. Then cast your Runes, and look up your answers in the Master Answer section. You'll find interpretations there for all your Work, Love, Money, and Strategy questions.

Another way to freestyle is to take advantage of the Index, which lists all of the questions used in the book. The Index will point you in the direction of a Reading that will answer the specific concern you have today. It may also suggest questions that you might want to ask.

CRAFT PROJECTS

Half the fun of using Runes is making them, and this book is loaded with Rune-making projects—ranging from simple to advanced. Just browse through the Extra, Extra Credit sections at the end of each Reading. I've test-driven them all, and they're a blast. All you need to get started is a scratch pad and a pen. The adventuresome can work their way up to power tools.

PARTY GAMES

Looking for something a little different for your next get-together with friends? Try Reading #16's Extra Credit section where the Runes will ask <u>you</u> the questions (!), in a friendly game of Truth or Dare. The Index lists other party games located throughout the book. And if you really want to get into it, practically any Reading in the book is fair game. You'll find your Runic horoscope in Reading #11. And for a talking board experience, try anagrams in Reading #20's Extra, Extra Credit section.

NUMBERS GAMES

For numbers hounds, *Runes in Ten Minutes* shows you various ways to use your Runes to get at numbers. For a numerological experience, follow the "Runeless" path noted above. To compute the odds that something will or won't happen, see the Extra Credit section of Reading #17. And—as a special bonus—here's a fun way to choose your lucky numbers for the next state lottery or church raffle:

To select winning numbers. This method works for any game that uses 40 numbers or less. To select your first number, mix up your Runes and ask: **What number will win for me in the drawing?** Reach into your Runes and select the one that feels most lucky. Note which Rune it is and whether it is upright or reversed. Then find it in this chart.

1	F	11	<	21	⋈	31	M
2	⌰	12	>	22	⋈	32	⋈
3	U	13	X	23	Y	33	⋈
4	⋂	14	⊬	24	⋏	34	Γ
5	⊦	15	⊲	25	S	35	⌡
6	⊣	16	H	26	↑	36	⋇
7	⊦	17	✝	27	↓	37	⋆
8	⋌	18	I	28	B	38	⋇
9	R	19	<>	29	⋜	39	⋈
10	⋋	20	⌁	30	M	40	◊

382

Presto, you've got your number. Jot it down, and place the Rune back in the pile. Draw another Rune to get the next number. And so on. If your game uses less than 40 numbers, remove the Runes you don't need before you make your picks. If you need a 40 (but not a zero), make Ⓞ worth 40. Keep drawing until you have all the numbers you need to play the game.

Your alphabet tiles will also serve you well for lucky-number draws. And the neat thing about them is that they accommodate games of 42, 44, or even 46 numbers. If you don't need all of the numbers in this chart, just remove the corresponding tiles before your draw.

1 Ⓕ	11 Ⓒ	21 Ⓐ	31 Ⓩ	41 Ⓛ
2 Ⓕ	12 Ⓒ	22 Ⓗ	32 Ⓢ	42 Ⓣ
3 Ⓤ	13 Ⓚ	23 Ⓝ	33 Ⓣ	43 Ⓧ
4 Ⓓ	14 Ⓚ	24 Ⓘ	34 Ⓘ	44 Ⓞ
5 Ⓣⓗ	15 Ⓠ	25 Ⓨ Ⓨ	35 Ⓑ	45 Ⓞ
6 Ⓣⓗ	16 Ⓞ	26 Ⓙ Ⓙ	36 Ⓖ	46 Ⓓ Ⓓ
7 Ⓐ	17 Ⓖ Ⓖ	27 Ⓔ Ⓔ	37 Ⓔ	0 Ⓞ
8 Ⓥ	18 Ⓦ	28 Ⓟ	38 Ⓔ	
9 Ⓡ	19 Ⓜ	29 Ⓙ	39 Ⓜ	
10 Ⓨ	20 Ⓥ	30 Ⓩ	40 Ⓦ	

To pick 3, just use the Runes that, upright or reversed, stand for the digits 0–9: Ⓞ, Ⓕ, Ⓤ, Ⓟ, Ⓐ, and Ⓡ (or use tiles Ⓞ, F, U, Th, A, and R). Mix up these six and select one. Consult the chart for your first digit. (There's only one trick: An R/Ⓡ upright or reversed counts either way as a 9.) Mix up all six Runes again, select your next Rune, and jot down your second digit. Repeat the process once more to get your third digit. **To pick 4,** just mix up these six Runes again and draw once more.

Since Runes were sometimes used to determine numbers, this is an authentic way to put them to use. Good luck in the drawing.

NAME GAMES

Runes were also originally used to write a person's name. And a number of the Readings in *Runes in Ten Minutes* are devoted to interpreting what the Runes in your name have to say about you. To get a full name analysis, conduct Readings #4, #5, #6, #7, #20, #21, #22, and #23.

GET LUCKY

Another authentic use of Runes is as good-luck charms. You will find the Rune that is exclusively yours in Reading #23. But you can use any Rune as an amulet. You might try using the one that turns up most frequently in your Readings. Or select any Rune that represents the virtues that you aspire to. Use the Master Answer section as a way of getting a feeling for which Rune might do the trick for you right now. Many New Age stores sell Rune pendants. Or you can just tuck one of your casting Runes in your pocket for good luck. (Don't forget to get it out the next time you consult.)

VISUALIZING THE RUNES

To help you visualize what each Rune stands for, *Runes in Ten Minutes* includes a "storybook" picture for each. Just turn to Readings #17, #18, and #19 to review them. The drawings that have been rendered for this book depict a fellow on his vision quest, since the idea of seeking your destiny is central in the Runes, and a wonderfully constructive way to use them. As a whole, *Runes in Ten Minutes* is designed to help you put the Runes to good use in your life.

. . . AND DON'T MISS THE EXTRA CREDITS

To get maximum value out of this book, do the Extra Credit sections! Most of them will give you an entirely different "trick" to do with the Reading you have just finished. Some of them even perform special tricks of their own! And a number of them will show you how to "gang up" three Readings into one—giving you even further mileage from your Runes. Taken all together, these "little extras" give you three books in one.

For Further Information

RECOMMENDED READING

If you'd like to read more about Runes and their rich and mysterious history, there are many fascinating books on the subject, but you might start with these . . .

Ralph Blum, *The Book of Runes*, St. Martin's Press, 1982, 1987. This is a great book for people who want to use their Runes for soul searching.

Robert M. Hoffstein, *A Mystical Key to the English Language*, Destiny Books, 1992. For alphabet-tile users, you'll find additional ways to interpret your English letters here.

R. I. Page, *Reading the Past: Runes*, British Museum Press, 1987. For a scholarly view on where Runes came from and what they were used for, this is a concise, authoritative, and informative overview.

Nigel Pennick, *Magical Alphabets*, Samuel Weiser, 1992. This is a fascinating book that not only talks about Runes, but about the mystical traditions surrounding other alphabets such as Hebrew and Greek.

Dr. James M. Peterson, *The Enchanted Alphabet*, Aquarian Press, 1988. This is an easily understandable general overview to the Runes, the mythology behind them, and the traditions surrounding them.

Edred Thorsson, *Rune Lore*, Samuel Weiser, 1987. For those who want to explore the history, philosophy, and especially the magical roots of Runes, there's no better source.

Donald Tyson, *Rune Magic*, Llewellyn, 1988. This is a charming book that focuses on the magical aspects of Runes in theory, history, and practice. A great read.

Index

ALL THE QUESTIONS YOU CAN ASK
(And everything else you can do)

With *Runes in Ten Minutes*, you can ask just about any question you like. The Index covers the questions that are specifically listed in the book. Scan the lists for those that will help you get at the issue on your mind today. Or turn to Reading #24 to learn how to frame your own questions. The Index also covers the other activities you can do and will point you down some of the paths you can take through the book.

INDEX TO ACTIVITIES

INDEX TO THE QUESTIONS

  * Extra Credit section
 ** Extra, Extra Credit section

DECISION MAKING

FAMILY, HOME, AND FRIENDS

 * Extra Credit section
** Extra, Extra Credit section

FAMILY, HOME, AND
FRIENDS (continued)   Reading

What is the lesson of my past homes?	3
What kind of love do I feel for my dog? my house?	19*
What will my children get from me?	5*
Where are my friends?	15
Where is this friendship headed?	15
Who are my true friends?	15
Who do I need to watch out for?	16
Who do I take after?	5
Who is my companion?	14

GENERAL QUESTIONS   Reading

How should I proceed with regard to _____?	3**
How's it going?	12*
Show me my options with regard to _____?	8*
Speak to me	12*
Spell out what I should know about _____.	20**
Tell me a tale about _____.	17
What are the odds I'll _____?	17*
What can I learn from _____?	13*
What do I need to watch out for?	16
What do I need?	10
What does _(so-and-so)_ see in me?	6*
What if I decide <u>not</u> to _____?	9
What if I decide to _____?	9
What if I do and what if I don't?	9*
What is the fate of _____?	23*
What is the lesson of my past?	3
What kind of a friend is _____?	15
What kind of love do I feel for my work? my art?	19*
What love will I know?	19*
What morals are involved in my decision?	20*
What must I do?	8
What should I do about _____?	3*
What will tomorrow bring?	2
What's meant to be?	23*

  * Extra Credit section
 ** Extra, Extra Credit section

* Extra Credit section
** Extra, Extra Credit section

LOVE, SEX, AND PASSION (continued)   *Reading #*

Will I be lucky in love?	1
Will she stand by me through and through? Will he?	14

LUCK   *Reading #*

Is this my lucky day?	1
What kind of luck will I have tomorrow?	1
When's the right day to buy a lottery ticket?	10*
Wishing stones	4**
Love charms	7*
Lucky charms	12**
Lucky numbers *(see Appendix)*	
Tree charms	8**

MONEY AND POWER   *Reading #*

How will everything turn out for the country?	2
Pretty please, give me some leads	21*
Tell me a bedtime story	17
What do I need?	10
What if I decide <u>not</u> to invest?	9
What is the fate of this investment?	23*
What is the fate of this political stand?	23*
What money will tomorrow bring?	2
What Runes do I need to do this deed?	22*
What's my secret with money?	7
Will I be lucky at achieving power?	1
Will I be lucky with money?	1

PERSONAL ASSESSMENT AND DEVELOPMENT   *Reading #*

How am I unique?	6
How can I remove the barriers to my progress?	18*
How lucky am I?	1
What are my charms?	6
What are my three best qualities?	6

   * Extra Credit section
 ** Extra, Extra Credit section

PLANNING, EVALUATION
AND FORECASTING   *Reading #*

 * Extra Credit section
** Extra, Extra Credit section

PLANNING, EVALUATION
AND FORECASTING (continued)   *Reading #*

What do I have going for me?	12*
What does the past add up to?	3
What if . . . ?	9
What is the fate of this project?	23*
What opposes me? my plans? my aspirations?	16
What powers will I need in the months ahead?	11*
What should I have learned from my past?	13*
What stage am I in?	12
What will tomorrow bring?	2
What's the word?	18
Where will I be at the end of the day?	19
Where will I wind up?	19
Will my luck hold out?	1
Yes/No	1*

QUICKIES   *Reading #*

Quick advice	3*
Thought for the day	23**
Words of advice	18

TIMING   *Reading #*

How's my timing?	10
Tell me when the moon is right	10**
Turn back the clock (correct a mistake)	13*
What will the coming year be like?	13
When will I know about this-or-that?	10**
When will such-and-such happen?	10**
When's the right day to _____?	10*

WORK AND CAREER   *Reading #*

How can I remove the barriers to my career plans?	18*
How should I proceed in my job hunt?	8
How will everything turn out for the company?	2

  * Extra Credit section
** Extra, Extra Credit section

INDEX TO RUNE FACTS AND FIGURES

 * Extra Credit section
** Extra, Extra Credit section

WHERE'S THAT CHART? (continued)   *Reading #*

* Extra Credit section
** Extra, Extra Credit section

INDEX TO RUNE LAYOUTS AND SPREADS

For an overview of layouts, see the Quick Reference Guide

 * Extra Credit section
** Extra, Extra Credit section

  * Extra Credit section
** Extra, Extra Credit section

Index

USING SPECIAL RUNES

CONDUCT THREE READINGS
AT ONCE

TRY OUT THE
MASTER ANSWER SECTION

* Extra Credit section
** Extra, Extra Credit section

Acknowledgments

Though this book was a joy to write . . . Runes also proved to be very demanding. I have virtually hundreds of recording artists to thank for keeping me company in the long nights. But this short list will have to suffice. Thanks to all of the poets and everyone who makes music, but especially . . .

Dr. Fiorella Terenzi, *Music from the Galaxies*, Island Records, 1991

    ◻   "Cosmic Time"

Rush, *Presto*, Atlantic Records, 1989

    ᚠ   "Red Tide"
    ᚺ   "Presto"
    ᛏ   "Anagram"

Loverboy, *Get Lucky*, Columbia Records, 1981

    ᚢ   "Lucky One"
    ᚾ   "Working for the Weekend"
    ᛒ   "Take Me to the Top"

Ozzy Osbourne, *No Rest for the Wicked*, Epic Records, 1988

    ᚦ   "Breaking All the Rules"
    ᛁ   "Miracle Man"
    ᛗ   "Fire in the Sky"

Aerosmith, *Get a Grip*, Geffen Records, 1993

    ᚦ   "Living on the Edge"
    ᛜ   "Cryin'"
    ᛗ   "Amazing"

Depeche Mode, *Songs of Faith and Devotion*, Sire Records, 1993

    ᚱ   "I Feel You"
    ᛇ   "One Caress"
    ᛚ   "Higher Love"

Madonna, *Erotica*, Sire Records, 1992

      <   "Rain"
      ᚴ   "Words"
      ᛝ   "Erotica"

Sting, *Ten Summoner's Tales*, A&M Records, 1993

      X   "Fields of Gold"
      Y   "Saint Augustine in Hell"
      ᚼ   "If I Ever Lose My Faith in You"

Guns N' Roses, *Use Your Illusion I*, Geffen Records, 1991

      ᚠ   "Don't Cry"
      ᛋ   "Live and Let Die"
      ᛗ   "November Rain"

Tom Capello, *The Lost Boys*, Original Motion Picture Soundtrack, Atlantic Records, 1987

      ᛟ   "I Still Believe"

For bringing me luck at the start, thanks to . . . INXS (*Welcome to Wherever You Are*), Bonnie Raitt (*Luck of the Draw*), Robert Palmer (*Addictions, Vol. I*), Jesus Jones (*Doubt*), Jon Bon Jovi (*Keep the Faith*), REM (*Automatic for the People*), and, as always, Madonna for "Like a Prayer."

For bringing me through the home stretch, deep gratitude to . . . Pearl Jam (*VS*), Bruce Cockburn (*Dart to the Heart*), and Meat Loaf (*Bat Out of Hell—II*).

With special thanks to Chris Miller at Avon Books.
No words can express . . .

And to Tory and Addie,
my two favorite Roonies.

M<
ᚠᛁᛏ<ᛁ
ᚱᛁᛋᛏ
ᚱᚢᛏᚠᛯ
ᚠᚠᚠᚠᚠᚠᚠᚠ

ek vitki rist runar

(AAAAAAAA)

Traditional Runic Inscription:
"I the magician carved these runes"

FASCINATING BOOKS OF SPIRITUALITY AND PSYCHIC DIVINATION

CLOUD NINE: A DREAMER'S DICTIONARY
by Sandra A. Thomson
77384-8/$6.99 US/$7.99 Can

SECRETS OF SHAMANISM: TAPPING THE SPIRIT POWER WITHIN YOU
by Jose Stevens, Ph.D. and Lena S. Stevens
75607-2/$5.99 US/$6.99 Can

TAROT IN TEN MINUTES
by R.T. Kaser
76689-2/$10.00 US/$12.00 Can

THE LOVERS' TAROT
by Robert Mueller, Ph.D., and Signe E. Echols, M.S., with Sandra A. Thomson
76886-0/$11.00 US/$13.00 Can

SEXUAL ASTROLOGY
by Marlene Masini Rathgeb
76888-7/$10.00 US/$12.00 Can